Occupational Medicine

Office Ergonomics

Guest Editor:

Martin Cherniack, MD, MPH
Director
Ergonomic Technology Center
University of Connecticut Health Center
Farmington, Connecticut

STATE OF THE ART REVIEWS

Volume 14/Number 1
HANLEY & BELFUS, INC.

January–March 1999
Philadelphia

Publisher: HANLEY & BELFUS, INC.
210 South 13th Street
Philadelphia, PA 19107
(215) 546-4995
Fax (215) 790-9330
Web site: http://www.hanleyandbelfus.com

OCCUPATIONAL MEDICINE: State of the Art Reviews is included in *Index Medicus, MEDLINE, BioSciences Information Service, Current Contents* and *ISI/BIOMED, CINAHL database, and Cumulative Index to Nursing & Allied Health Literature.*

OCCUPATIONAL MEDICINE: State of the Art Reviews   ISSN 0885-114X
January–March 1999   Volume 14, Number 1   ISBN 1-56053-285-8

OCCUPATIONAL MEDICINE: State of the Art Reviews is published quarterly by Hanley & Belfus, Inc., 210 South 13th Street, Philadelphia, Pennsylvania 19107. Periodical postage paid at Philadelphia, PA, and at additional mailing offices.

POSTMASTER: Send address changes to OCCUPATIONAL MEDICINE: State of the Art Reviews, Hanley & Belfus, Inc., 210 South 13th Street, Philadelphia, PA 19107.

The 1999 subscription price is $92.00 per year U.S., $102.00 outside U.S. (add $40.00 for air mail).

Occupational Medicine: State of the Art Reviews
Vol. 14, No. 1, January–March 1999

OFFICE ERGONOMICS
Martin Cherniack, MD, MPH, Editor

CONTENTS

CONTRIBUTORS

Benjamin C. Amick, III, PhD
Research Scientist, The Health Institute, New England Medical Center; Lecturer, Department of Environmental and Occupational Medicine, Harvard University School of Public Health; Assistant Professor, Department of Family Medicine and Community Health, Tufts University School of Medicine, Boston, Massachusetts. Adjunct Scientist, Institute for Work and Health, Ontario, Canada

Ulf O.V. Bergqvist, DrMedSci, MSciTech
Researcher, Department of Occupational Health, National Institute for Working Life, Solna, Sweden

Robert F. Bettendorf, BBA
President, The Institute for Office Ergonomics, Manchester Center, Vermont

Stephen Burastero, MD

Hong Chang, PhD
Statistician, The Health Institute, New England Medical Center, Boston, Massachusetts

Martin Cherniack, MD, MPH
Professor of Medicine, Ergonomic Technology Center, Division of Occupational and Environmental Medicine, University of Connecticut Health Center, Farmington, Connecticut

Allard E. Dembe, ScD
Assistant Professor, Department of Family Medicine and Community Health, University of Massachusetts Medical School, Worcester, Massachusetts

Richard Townsend Gun, MBBS, FAFOM (RACP)
Senior Lecturer in Occupational and Environmental Health, Department of Public Health, University of Adelaide, Adelaide, South Australia

Peter Tomas Jezukaitis, MBBS, FAFOM (RACP)
Occupational Physician, Tusmore, South Australia

Charles Levenstein, PhD, MSOH
Professor of Work Environment Policy, Work Environment Department, University of Massachusetts, Lowell, Massachusetts

Susan E. Mackinnon, MD
Shoenberg Professor of Surgery and Chief, Division of Plastic and Reconstructive Surgery, Washington University School of Medicine, St. Louis; Plastic Surgeon-in-Chief, Barnes-Jewish Hospital, St. Louis, Missouri

Tim F. Morse, PhD
Assistant Professor, Department of Community Medicine, Ergonomic Technology Center, University of Connecticut Health Center, Farmington, Connecticut

Ivan G. Most, ScD
President, Strategic Occupational Health Management, Inc., Cape Elizabeth, Maine

Christine B. Novak, PT
Research Assistant Professor, Division of Plastic and Reconstructive Surgery, Washington University School of Medicine, St. Louis, Missouri

Emil F. Pascarelli, MD
Professor of Clinical Medicine, Department of Medicine, Columbia University College of Physicians and Surgeons, New York, New York

Laura Punnett, ScD
Professor, Department of Work Environment, University of Massachusetts Lowell, Lowell, Massachusetts

Pat Tittiranonda, PhD, MPH
Post Doctoral Fellow and Ergonomist, Interdisciplinary Ergonomics Research Program, Health Services, University of California, Lawrence Livermore National Laboratory, Livermore, California

David Rempel, MD
Associate Professor, Department of Medicine, University of California, San Francisco, California

Naomi G. Swanson, PhD

Nicholas Warren, ScD
Assistant Professor of Medicine, Ergonomic Technology Center, Division of Occupational and Environmental Medicine, University of Connecticut Health Center, Farmington, Connecticut

1999 ISSUES

Office Ergonomics
Edited by Martin Cherniack, MD, MPH
University of Connecticut
Farmington, Connecticut
Animal Handlers
Edited by Ricky L. Langley, MD, MPH
Kernodle Clinic
Burlington, North Carolina

Special Populations
Edited by Howard Frumkin, MD
Emory University
Atlanta, Georgia
and Glenn Pransky, MD, MOccH
University of Massachusetts
Worcester, Massachusetts
Plastics and Rubber Industries
Edited by Richard Lewis, MD, MPH
University of Louisville
Louisville, Kentucky

1998 ISSUES

Low Back Pain
Edited by Gerard A. Malanga, MD
University of Medicine and Dentistry
of New Jersey
Newark, New Jersey
Workers' Compensation
Edited by T. L. Guidotti, MD, MPH
University of Alberta
Edmonton, Alberta, Canada
and John W. F. Cowell, MD, Msc
Workers' Compensation Board of Alberta
Edmonton, Alberta, Canada

Hand and Upper Extremity Injuries
Edited by Morton L. Kasdan, MD
University of Louisville
Louisville, Kentucky
and V. Jane Derebery, MD
Concentra Medical Center
Austin Texas
Managed Care
Edited by Jeffrey S. Harris, MD, MPH,
  MBA
J. Harris Associates, Inc.
Mill Valley, California

1997 ISSUES

The Pharmaceutical Industry
Edited by Gregg M. Stave, MD, JD, MPH
Glaxo Wellcome Inc.
Research Triangle Park, North Carolina
and Ron Joines, MD, MPH
SmithKline Beecham
Philadelphia, Pennsylvania
Human Health Effects of Pesticides
Edited by Matthew C. Keifer, MD, MPH
Harborview Medical Center
Seattle, Washington

Diagnostic Testing
Edited by Michael H. LeWitt, MD
Great Valley Health
Paoli, Pennsylvania
The Health Care Worker
Edited by Melissa A. McDiarmid, MD, MPH
University of Maryland
Baltimore, Maryland
and Ellen Kessler, MD, MPH
INOVA Fairfax Hospital
Falls Church, Virginia

Ordering Information:
Subscriptions for full year and single issues are available from the publishers—
Hanley & Belfus, Inc., 210 South 13th Street, Philadelphia, PA 19107
Telephone (215) 546-7293; (800) 962-1892. Fax (215) 790-9330.

PREFACE

The digitalization of traditional office work and the introduction of computer-related technologies to diverse work sites and processes represents a phase of technological substitution that may well define a historic period. It recapitulates in scope the last century's introduction of petroleum by vertically transforming work processes and also linking them in new ways. This *Occupational Medicine: State of the Art Reviews*, entitled *Office Ergonomics*, has twin objectives: (1) to examine a nontraditional class of upper extremity disorders that have been associated with office work, and (2) to present an approach to the identification and weighting of multiple worksite factors, including the impact of devices and furniture, work organization, underlying physical predisposition and risk, and the psychosocial milieu. From this perspective, *Office Ergonomics* outlines an approach to problem solving that departs from the traditional occupational medicine model, in which precise exposure quantification, uniform case definition, and determination of thresholds for dose-response relationships have been hallmarks of effective hazard control.

In their overview chapter, "Risk Factors for Musculoskeletal Disorders Among Computer Users," Tittiranonda, Burastero, and Rempel describe soft tissue symptoms and disorders associated with devices that in less than two decades have become as common as the desktop telephone. Allard Dembe's "The Changing Nature of Office Work: Effects on Repetitive Strain Injuries" poses a broader perspective, characterizing the electronic office within a two-century process of industrialization, thus recalling that changes in work organization and cultural and social transformation have an older pedigree than device introduction, and that the relationship of technological change to physical disease is rarely one-dimensional. In some respects, the development of the modern office represents an eclipse of physical labor by intellectual labor and the potential for individual worker autonomy over managerial hierarchy. When viewed from the looking glass of the explosive mines and infested workshops that were the domain of the 19th century founders of modern occupational medicine, the electronic workplace represents a stage of considerable progress. Ergonomics, with the potential to anticipate human comfort as well as performance, poses an alternative to process engineering. But the expectations of the Enlightenment and the optimism of 19th century Socialism have been satisfied by a very equivocal type of workplace freedom.

Well-being in the office has shifted, in part, from questions of wages, hours, and lethal inhalation to subtler concerns over physical health and its relationship to work organization and the psychosocial milieu. The public and professional recognition of acquired neuromuscular and musculoskeletal diseases, induced or aggravated by the workplace, has caused a graduated attention to workplace organization and equipment—the field of office ergonomics—as well as a reactive skepticism. Why should activities that require modest outputs of muscle force, compared with traditional agriculture, manufacturing, and domestic labor, produce broad public concern, significant reports of disease, and a professionalized corrective response? Robert Bettendorf's chapter, "A Low-Cost, Effective Approach to Office Ergonomics," raises an intriguing consideration. If 90% of individual worksite evaluations at a major corporation lead to recommendations for modification, albeit low-cost modification, are the formulaic hazard-response and surveillance models that prevail in occupational medicine sufficient for the modern office? A reflexive skepticism could conclude that a stirring call for continuous organizational reform and anticipatory review of introduced technology only rationalizes the specialization of professional ergonomists, thus socializing an academic discipline whose recommendations are not necessarily accessible to rigorous evaluation. However, the contributions by Ivan Most, Nick Warren and I, and Robert Bettendorf suggest another direction, already empirically applied. A democratized process of effective worksite review involving worker, manager, and scientific professional *has produced effective interventions, reduced injury, and raised job satisfaction.*

A few things should be said about the organization of this issue. Although a singular and specialized topic such as office ergonomics seems sufficiently narrow, there are still potentially restrictive latitudes. There was a basic choice between emphasizing breadth (the review feature) or emphasizing selective current issues and controversies (the state of the art feature). This volume tends strongly toward the latter approach. Because a focus on the most current scientific work risks the recruitment of unconnected contributions, important areas involving the basic sciences have been deemphasized or omitted. Accordingly, while some of the most interesting recent work has been in the areas of biomechanical modeling of activity-related musculoskeletal and neuromuscular upper extremity disorders and in the measurement of movement dynamics, neither of these areas is reviewed in this volume. Similarly, basic science approaches to muscle physiology and gene expression and to subclinical injury to muscle and tendon have been left out. While the chapters by Novak and Mackinnon and by Pascarelli deal with clinical considerations, including etiology, diagnosis, and medical management, this volume is not primarily a clinical compilation.

There are several chapters which establish a broad context for *Office Ergonomics,* "Risk Factors for Musculoskeletal Disorders Among Computer Users" presents a balanced and conventional synopsis of the most common disorders and generally recognized substantive studies on office ergonomics. Physical factors, including typing speed, work-rest cycles, and non-neutral joint postures, and personal factors, such as gender and anthropometry, are discussed, along with work organization and psychosocial factors. The observations that sustained awkward postures, duration of computer use, and work organization factors have been consistently associated with soft tissue disorders among office workers, and that etiology involves multiple factors, is a consensual starting point for this volume. Novak and MacKinnon present an individually centered view of the contributions of dynamic posture and soft tissue and skeletal adaptation to clinical symptoms in the computer-using population. This view is an extension of anthropometrics but also poses a conceptual alternative to fixed architectural nerve entrapment models that have developed from surgical observation. Tim Morse's contribution, "Surveillance and the Problems of Assessing Office-Related Injury," completes the overview portion of this volume. On the one hand he offers an informed primer on the different available reporting systems; on the other, he explores impediments to early reporting and active surveillance that involve social and economic presumptions as well as mechanistic difficulties.

In a more specialized historical contribution, Allard Dembe charts the evolution of the modern office from the 1880s, documenting the ongoing feminization of office work and the episodic nature of the introduction of new technologies. He notes that recognized risk factors in office work—awkward postures, routinized work, time pressures, organizational factors—apply to other domains of employment and that work-associated musculoskeletal disease has been documented by occupational physicians throughout the past two centuries, preceding the introduction of the video display terminal. He delineates the contributions of political and cultural life to disease recognition and acceptance. In a somewhat complementary chapter, Richie Gun and P.T. Jezukaitis write from the Australian homeland of the repetitive strain injury epidemic and differentiate between the politically influenced acceptance and relegation of office-related upper extremity disease and a less mercurial evolution of understanding of soft tissue ergonomics and pain syndromes.

Benjamin Amick, Naomi Swanson, and Hong Chang, in "Office Technology and Musculoskeletal Disorders: Building an Ecological Model," offer an ecological model that applies path analysis to the interplay of physical factors, work organization, and healthcare use. In evaluating the role of psychosocial variables and work organization, they generate both surprising and intriguing results: (1) health care utilization appears much more significantly driven by symptom severity than by underlying mental health or individual traits, and (2) the structure of work organization is more predictive of musculoskeletal disorders than dose estimates based on simple time at the keyboard. Nick Warren and I, in our chapter "Ambiguities in Office-Related Injury: The Poverty of Present Approaches," address the arena of multifactorial risk from another perspective. We juxtapose the complexity of a research environment, which must move between molecular mechanisms of disease and group surveys, and the very active culture of empirical ergonomic intervention against a surprisingly stubborn and sometimes ideological debate over first cause. Laura Punnett and Ulf Bergqvist continue the themes of psychosocial and work organizational factors introduced by Amick, Swanson, and Chang by looking selectively at gender issues in the office environment. Ivan Most takes these considerations involving work organization to a more applied level by exploring a specific organizational culture in a large New England employer and charting the impacts of strategic ergonomic intervention. Robert Bettendorf offers a more general approach to developing an ergonomic problem-solving program. He also distinguishes between uncertainties that are the focus of research and the introduction of corrective measures that are accepted and, most importantly, work.

This volume concludes with the contributions of Emil Pascarelli and Charles Levenstein, who provide a social and economic perspective. Pascarelli makes it clear that treatment and intervention do not occur in an aseptic and fully controllable world of corridors and office dividers. The existing worker's compensation system and the evolving system of managed care define both the limits and sequence of injury management. Levenstein attempts a micro-economic analysis of the impacts of office injury, based principally on data from the State of New York. While the assessment of direct and indirect costs may have circumscribed utility for the individual worksite, he offers an approach that is highly accessible for policy and planning.

The approaches presented in *Office Ergonomics* pose several clinical, organizational, and conceptual challenges to practitioners of occupational medicine. Descriptive terms for upper arm syndromes, such as repetitive strain injury, cumulative trauma disorders, work-related musculoskeletal disorders, and even carpal tunnel syndrome and thoracic outlet syndrome, are only partially illuminated by differentiating between "hard" disorders, such as entrapment disorders, and "softer" pain and functional conditions that affect office workers. Because the electronic office imposes some standardization of devices and operations, variations in exposure or extrinsic risk factors arise in large part from work organization. Traditionally, the organization of work has fallen outside of the purview of regulatory occupational medicine, and the notion of administrative control fails utterly to address the connections between organizational and task structure and human performance and workplace well being. For all of these reasons, the notions of measured dose and target organ are insufficient. The terms "ecology of disease" and "wholism" creep into this volume because cognition, work organization and culture, and internal or intrinsic styles of work and activity all complement the movement and response of nerves, muscles, and tendons. Occupational medicine has always required expansive and integrated skills of its best practitioners. The modern office still requires these qualifications.

Martin Cherniack, MD, MPH
GUEST EDITOR

MARTIN CHERNIACK, MD, MPH
NICK WARREN, ScD

AMBIGUITIES IN OFFICE-RELATED INJURY: THE POVERTY OF PRESENT APPROACHES

From the Ergonomic Technology
  Center
University of Connecticut Health
  Center
Farmington, Connecticut

Reprint requests to:
Martin Cherniack, MD, MPH
Ergonomic Technology Center
University of Connecticut Health
  Center
263 Farmington Avenue
Farmington, CT 06030-6210

Acquired injuries of the upper extremity, associated with the modern office, have generated a curious set of controversies. There is basic disagreement over what to properly call these disorders and fundamental skepticism about their existence and significance. From another perspective, there is a track record of highly successful workplace intervention and a deepening eclectic body of investigative work that encompasses the physiology of muscle dynamics, group psychology and work organization, and the neurobiology of complex task performance. This chapter explores scientific and procedural perspectives that have evolved around the characterization of upper extremity disorders in the contemporary office. While ambiguous terminology and diffuse scientific characterizations are shared with other branches of medicine and public health, these disorders also challenge more traditional notions of occupational disease, wherein duplicable exposure measurement, specific clinical syndromes, and elimination of risk are the subsoil of methodologic approaches. The overlap of cognitive and physical tasks, the interaction between external and intrinsic risk factors, the diversity of relative exposures, and a notion of well being that is cognitive, emotional, and physical all come into play around office-related upper extremity problems. There is ample terrain for creative integration across technical fields and for confusion.

In fewer than 20 years, electronic workstations and keyboard data entry have become so interwoven with industrial and office work that they are now fundamental job requirements. The concomitant rise in upper extremity symptoms associated with the evolving electronic office has been precipitous. From one perspective, these are mundane and clinically familiar pain disorders—a spectrum of work-related musculoskeletal problems occurring in a new key and meriting accurate medical diagnoses.[27] From another point of view, they are not true diseases but reactive phenomena, requiring a sociologic and psychological metric. Such socially determined somatic manifestations are inappropriately linked to workplace risks by crude diagnostics and faulty epidemiologic technique. From this viewpoint, medical reductionism of office-related symptoms to a taxonomy of anatomic syndromes and tissue-specific diagnoses is a poor approach to disease characterization.[40] These opposing explanatory models for upper extremity symptoms in the office persist with both an impressive and surprising resilience. The disagreement over the existence of an association between electronic office work and upper extremity symptoms is frequently antagonistic but, now in its second decade, is no longer novel. For more than 3 years, the *American Journal of Hand Surgery* has printed an ongoing exchange of descriptive articles, letters to the editors, and editorials on the subject, underscoring the very basic and refractory nature of this peculiar controversy.[49] Medical controversies, driven by intervention trials and empirical results, usually tend either toward acceptance of a prevailing model or a recasting of the scientific questions. That upper extremity problems in the office should continue to stimulate a fundamental debate is odd for another reason. One of the particular characteristics of upper extremity disorders in the office workplace is the lingering and intense debate over definitions and causation of disease when large portions of the field have clearly moved on to a more detailed level of laboratory study, clinical intervention, and organizational approaches to control. Despite the academic debate, both private and public sectors are well advanced in the pursuit of empirical solutions, some seemingly quite effective.

POPULATION-BASED RESEARCH ANOMALIES

A legitimate platform for divergent perspectives on upper extremity symptoms in the office comes from piecemeal and sometimes contradictory evidence arising from population-based observational research. One of the most demonstrative of the numerous examples is the geographic selectivity that was a feature of the first concentrated outbreak of office-related symptoms in Australia. The high prevalence of symptoms in public sector workers in New South Wales and Victoria was not duplicated in employees engaged in seemingly identical processes in Queensland and South Australia.[24,45,51] A persistent contrarian interpretation has been that these anatomically nonspecific acquired pain syndromes, called repetitive strain injury (RSI), were the product of altered medical sensibilities and popular suggestion rather than a new or computer-specific disease.[33] Clinical observers, more impressed with the consistent patterns of symptoms associated with work at the electronic workstation, have noted another aspect of geographic selectivity: the discordance between the public and professional attention paid to upper extremity symptoms in office workers.[17,50] In some quarters, the electronic keyboard symbolizes the entire field of ergonomics. Nevertheless, office-related disorders demonstrate a relatively modest prevalence of work-related lost-time injury compared to soft tissue disorders in other job categories[12] (see Tim Morse's chapter for a more detailed analysis performed on Connecticut Workers' Compensation data). The adage that newspapermen are in the first place correspondents of their own experience is reflected in the attention paid to keyboard-related problems that affect the newsroom. There has been special, perhaps disproportionate, emphasis in several national studies of injuries among newspaper personnel.[30,57] While it is likely that the technological transformation of the newsroom explains some of this emphasis, there is also the irresistible power of firsthand experience. The issue has already become somewhat historical: descriptions of symptoms proliferate in other work settings.[9]

The regionally disparate nature of early reporting patterns is not exceptional and usually reflects some combination of concentrated susceptible populations and proximate and attuned medical surveillance mechanisms. The 1981 literature on the human immunodeficiency virus is a recent example of an unfolding pattern of case- and then population-based disease recognition. The initial reports from Los Angeles, San Francisco, and New York suggested a coastal pattern of disease. However, this notion of a New York-Los Angeles-San Francisco axis of disease was supplanted by better explanations as the disease vector was characterized.

Moreover, broadening clinical recognition does not necessarily coincide with severity or attack rate. Reports of acquired upper extremity disorders in shipyard workers[43] and in symphony orchestra members[26] exceed those in newspaper workers in severity and prevalence but have earned considerably less attention. The recognition of disease severity is complex, multicentric, and unfair if fairness is gauged in proportion to the extent of pathology and adverse impact on daily life. Whatever may be attributable to cultural sensitivities toward and presumptions about a disease, there is nothing particularly unique about the appearance of episodic and inconsistent epidemiologic patterns with the recognition of a new disease. The same is true for cumbersome disease acronyms that persist after new information on the biologic mechanism has rendered the acronym obsolete. The early accounts of the AIDS epidemic entailed highly inaccurate suppositions on cause and an enduring acronym that no longer encompasses biologic understanding.

Substantial confusion arises due to the linking of symptom patterns to unsatisfactory acronyms, such as CTD (cumulative trauma disorders), RSI, WRMSD (work-related musculoskeletal disorders, and WRUED (work-related upper extremity disorders). Upper extremity pain can occur in office jobs involving little repetition and lacking an immediately observable temporal sequence of exposure and outcome that is usually associated with the notion of "injury." Armstrong et al. have presented a valuable working model for the development of upper extremity and neck disorders that invokes the interrelated variables of external exposures, internal dose, body capacity, and body response.[4] However, the notion of accumulation of trauma implies overwhelming of a threshold of repair by chronic exposure, a model perhaps more appropriate for cadmium or lead toxicity than keyboarding. A sequence of excessive effort and insufficient repair time, implicit in the idea of "overuse," seems sensible but is uncomfortably metaphoric. Issues around the dynamic assessment of muscle and tendon physiology are complex, and there is nothing simple or straightforward about the generation of practical prohibitions in the office environment where extrinsic factors do not extend physical capacity, as conventionally measured.

LIMITATIONS OF BIOMECHANICAL CONCEPTS FOR POPULATION-BASED AND MEDICAL APPLICATIONS

Gait laboratories have produced a relatively restricted vocabulary and set of methods for characterizing congenital and acquired movement disorders of the lower extremity.[19,20] This concision has been valuable to a relatively small community of biomechanists and orthopedic surgeons, but the arena of these practitioners largely excludes workplace and environmental associations and attribution related to aging. Biomechanical language often suffers in translation from the laboratory to clinical and epidemiologic usage. The obvious and global presence of redundantly cycled tasks in computer work, and the usual absence of single provocative events for acquired upper extremity symptoms in office workers, has drawn attention to the repetitive character of electronic keyboarding.[5] This biodynamic consideration is a departure from the emphasis in low back disease, the essential musculoskeletal disorder. Low back disease in the workplace has been studied and regulated in relation to heavy lifting and loading forces.[38,39] By contrast, there is a plausible analogy to office-related arm problems in heavy industry, where increased upper extremity symptoms are associated with short cycling times for redundant tasks (less than 30 seconds). These tasks can be legitimately characterized as repetitive work.[60,63]

The effort to develop an acceptable generalizing acronym for upper extremity, neck, and shoulder problems in the office population incorporates these dynamic assumptions. There is RSI, CTD, repetitive motion disorder (RMD), and overuse syndrome. The often acrimonious arguments over the accuracy of these terms are well known. Controversies of terminology aside, assigning a quantifiable threshold for repetition in the office environment is both elusive and complex. Telephone operators, airline reservation clerks, and inventory specialists may perform fewer than 10,000 keystrokes in a workday, but their shift may be spent in a sedentary posture at a poorly designed workstation. Dedicated word processing and data entry involving the same type of workstation postures may require more than 150,000 keystrokes per day. Stratification in exposure assessment is an obvious problem.

The uncertainty associated with identifying common biodynamic risk factors in the office workplace merges with a more fundamental problem: acquired pain syndromes and soft tissue disorders lack an obligate association with one specific work process or task. Hadler takes issue with the association of a tissue-based disease and work processes.[29] He observes that we do not refer to angina as "stairclimbers' chest," thus differentiating between pain that is intermittent, nonspecific, and serendipitously associated with an external event and a tissue-based pathology that can be reliably associated with an internal mechanism of disease. This analogy, too, is simplistic and avoids a much larger issue. A default to a common cache of symptoms or pathology that eschews etiology also can be inexact. A homogenizing term that incorporates multiple diagnoses associated with a complex and changing work environment might seem to offer a more enduring application than seamstress' cramp, telegrapher's cramp, stenographer's hand, or IBM user's regional myofasciitis. Miner's phthisis has a more localized context than the more universalizing silicosis or pneumoconiosis, but the latter terms hardly capture the sophisticated disease mechanism that is pursued in current silica research. Disease terminology abounds with language that now seems too local or episodic, that is diffuse and inconclusive, or that recalls an archaic disease process. Ischemic heart disease includes symptoms and altered physiology and, on a more basic level, patterns of vascular response that are the index of pharmacologic intervention. Its inherent imprecision does not diminish the utility of the term, and two generations of clinical research have not extinguished competing universalizing descriptive terms: coronary heart disease and coronary artery disease.

Calling arm symptoms "extensor carpi ulnaris tendinitis associated with data entry" or "input device-related medial epicondylitis localized to the flexor insertion" does not mean that a loose and metamorphic term such as cumulative trauma disorder has been replaced with satisfactory anatomic precision. Clinicians rightly regard epicondylitis and tendinitis as broad and imprecise symptom categories rather than tissue-specific diagnoses. Some observers have differentiated between diagnoses attributable to specific anatomy (such as DeQuervain's, or first dorsal compartment syndrome) and more diffuse cramps or focal dystonias and musculotendinous pain.[18] However, even this more deliberate dichotomy offers only limited additional precision. Diagnoses such as carpal tunnel syndrome (CTS) are highly problematic compilations of signs and symptoms; similar quantitative test results may homogenize quite different pathologies and therefore suggest treatments that are very industry- or process-specific. The apparent extrinsic nerve compressions in meatpackers,[52] and vibration-related polyneuropathy in foresters,[22] have differing etiologies and manifestations that undermine the usefulness of a single category of compression neuropathy or the comparison of results on nerve conduction tests.[41] The lack of a straightforward anatomic reference may reflect the underdevelopment of an appropriate disease model or reflect that there are similar clinical endpoints with overlapping or homologous features, but also with different underlying pathologies. The point is that the arguments over best terminology are probably unsolvable because descriptive terms serve various purposes. The coexistence of a broad descriptive category for enclosing multiple diagnoses, more specific tissue-based ICD-9 diagnoses, and then more scientific descriptive diagnoses should not be disturbing. In the diagnosis and treatment of soft tissue disorders, there are often multiple sites of symptom expression and tissue involvement that override single-site diagnoses. The association between proximal low back and hip disorders and ankle and foot disorders is a cornerstone of lower extremity rehabilitation. If generalizing terms are used as a shorthand, their use does not imply that more specific pathology is being ignored. Descriptive terms such as RSI or distal hand pain in the office are functionally misleading only if the shorthand becomes a substitute for pursuing different underlying mechanisms. But the limitation of broadly inclusive terminology has as its mirror image the limitation of grouping disparate and unconnected risks. The elusiveness of diagnoses has much less to do with the inadequacy of the descriptive language than with the fact that these are highly complex conditions that strain our capacity to measure tissue response and the dynamic interplay of cognitive, physiologic, and external factors. One danger is that the grouping of complex factors into broad categories of risk can appear to enclose most of the major parameters of disease causation, when the individual factors may be insufficiently quantified. This is an altogether different sensibility than a refusal to consider the relationship between acquired or exacerbated pain and discomfort and work processes.

DISEASE DEFINITION, WORK-RELATEDNESS, AND SOCIAL CONTEXT

The very different conventions used to describe injuries to musicians and artists provides another context for appreciating the controversy surrounding upper extremity disorders in office workers. Over the past two decades, acquired musculotendinous and neuromuscular disorders of the upper extremity, sometimes called overuse syndrome, have been recognized as a particular hazard for performing artists, especially for musicians.[11] From these clinical observations, generally collected by hand surgeons, distinctive patterns of high-performance posture and technique have been identified. These include ulnar nerve compression and flexor carpi ulnaris inflammation in pianists with effective dysfunction of the fourth and fifth fingers, and problems in the dorsal vibrato hand compartments of string players, reflecting mechanically inefficient hyperextension and flexor shortening.[42,44] Fifth-finger problems in flutists related to key location represent another common disorder.[16] Upper extremity problems in musicians include a range of anatomically distinct and functional problems—associated with a specific array of postures particular to individual instruments—that have raised attention in the last decade. The literature on upper extremity disorders in musicians uses descriptive terms, such as dystonic flexion,[16] hand and wrist disorders in musicians,[1] musical hands,[47] overuse syndrome in musicians,[46] or, simply, hand and wrist injuries in performing artists.[11] Similarly, in the growing field of sports medicine, the terms "sports injuries" and "sports-related injuries" are usually accepted even though patients often are not professional or amateur sportsmen, and treatment addresses both acute on-field injuries and acquired wear-and-tear diseases. How are these differing perspectives to be explained?

Some of the ambiguity and controversy over positing work-relatedness in office disorders appears to have an administrative origin, even though, in principle, workers' compensation plans do not differentiate between diseases induced purely by an exposure, underlying proclivities that may be brought over a symptom threshold by office tasks, or mild chronic symptoms that are amplified to a point of painful function or dysfunction. It seems likely that the performance skills of athletes and musicians are more highly prized than those of office workers, and pathology tends to be more respected and attributed to individual effort and self-discipline. Sports medicine addresses the injuries of a younger and generally well-insured population. Conversely, musicians are often not well covered by health insurance, infrequently use workers' compensation systems, and often go without treatment. Because of workers' compensation, potential federal regulations, and intervention costs, issues of causality and liability are more likely to be disputed in office-based disorders. An ideological objection to assumptions of work-relatedness is poorly represented by arguments over biologic mechanism.

Another important barrier to disease recognition and control involves the interplay between personal (or intrinsic) causes of disease and extrinsic equipment and processes at work. We do not commonly think of the violin or the tennis racket as sources of exposure or as unsafe tools, but superior designs from the perspective of health effects have been proposed and would have some advantages. Just like industrial tools, instruments and sports equipment can be reengineered to reduce the extrinsic stressors on soft tissues. Instead, there is an acceptance that technique and a fortunate or reinforced anatomy are essential components of performance. Tradition and the pursuits of performance mitigate against major equipment modification. The importance of technique variation, personal conditioning, anthropometric factors, and individual skill and intelligence are only too obvious when comparing the effortless playing of complex music with the efforts of a music student with a contracted left hand and painful wrists.

The recognition of a more complex interaction between work and individual is particularly susceptible to the challenges of ideology and social sensitivity. The workplace can be understood as a ubiquitous daily presence with an impact on many acquired diseases. From a different perspective, practitioners may consider the problem of occupational disease solved when purely extrinsic exposures have been contained or eliminated. In 1977, Hadler wrote:

> *We are not studying diseases of industries but of individuals. What is at issue is not whether people who work in mines, foundries, banks, etc., have diseases, but what particular pattern of usage is associated with a particular sample of clinical pathology. NIOSH* [National Institute for Safety and Health] *has the responsibility to perform research for the purpose of recommending safety and health standards. Perhaps a de-*

tailed understanding of the influence of pattern of usage on the pattern of disease would prove as useful to NIOSH in approaching its goal as to physicians faced with the clinical dilemmas of these diseases.

Twenty years later, the same writer stated the other side of this proposition with equivalent succinctness[29]:

Regional musculoskeletal disorders are a part of life. The likelihood of experiencing such morbidity is not a function of physical exposure for the wide range of exposures in the many industrial settings that have been studied. In these settings, regional musculoskeletal disorders represent a challenge in coping for the worker who is hurting and a challenge for management to eliminate barriers to coping.

Regardless of whether the author's own thinking has evolved, there have been profound changes in the culture of work in the intervening 20 years. In 1977 the common characteristics of pathology and acquired pain and discomfort associated with patterns of use were filtered through the fabric of the existing American industrial workplace with its tradition of indifference to public regulation. In 1997, the terrain has shifted to less tolerance of routine discomfort and disabling injury. With the aging of the workforce and the extension of civil rights to disability, a sensitivity to a broader concept of disability is evolving in large portions of the private sector, as it has in the public sector.

An additional problem in assigning a work-related etiology is the ubiquity of degenerative musculoskeletal change across all sectors of the population. The classic comparison can be made with the high frequency of low back pain and degenerative spinal disease.[53,65] Traumatic arthritis is certainly relevant to carpometacarpal pain or posttraumatic injury in athletes, but it appears to be less pertinent in the office population. The traumatic injury model suggests strong temporal and causative links between injury and long-term symptoms. Accumulated injury and gradual change in joints has a less direct link. By comparison, epicondylitis is relatively uncommon in the general population given the plurality of degenerative elbow disease in the population at autopsy.[15] Medial epicondylar symptoms are unusually common in the office population, and they appear at a younger age than in the general population.[6] These may not be the same injuries that we have observed in athletes. The discordance between altered image tissue architecture and symptoms is more a feature of age-related dysfunction or gradually acquired pain syndromes than of subacute injury.

ERGONOMICS AS A SEMANTIC PROBLEM

A semantic problem with more widespread consequences arises when "ergonomics" is used as an encompassing term to describe methods transferred from biomechanics to occupational medicine. The more traditional applications of ergonomics to human factors have strong bases in experimental psychology, perception, and design. On the other hand, to control population-based effects occupational health has relied heavily on the quantification of exposures and their regulation. The notions of an extrinsic exposure, a body-moderated dose, and a response by an "unskilled" organ or tissue does not carry over to the industrial and office workplace. While muscles and nerves are relatively uncomplicated compared to livers and lungs, the tasks of violinists and data processors are complex, relying on learned sequences of response and often on the translation of sophisticated ideas into a work process. Martin et al. point out that typing involves complex, often "programmed" coordination of large numbers of muscles.[48] Once learned, these programs serve the same function as "macros" on a computer keyboard: a complex set of movements can be efficiently performed with minimal conscious attention and with reduced need for sensory feedback. This is important because the short delays of the electronic keyboard (< 100 msec) are too brief to involve proprioceptive and reflex-derived responses.

A fully realized ergonomics approach addresses the interrelationship between a thinking worker, specific neuromusculature, a device or apparatus, and the physical and psychosocial environment in which the task is performed. But an impoverished and primarily extrinsic concept of effective exposure persists in the field. Hadler is not alone in using the term "ergonomic exposure" to tether a conventional notion of graded extrinsic exposure to processes in the electronic office.[29] NIOSH has introduced the concept of a traumatogen in mimicry of an exposure model in which the extrinsic component is quantifiable in units. Some mechanical or physical factors encountered at work, such as segmental vibration, lighting, temperature extremes, and mechanical compression of tissues are exposures in this limited sense. For instance, while biomechanical factors may reduce or exacerbate the effects of vibration exposure to varying degrees, and the response physiology is incompletely understood, a stationary bench grinder and a pneumatic burr machine will produce the same patterns of Raynaud's phenomenon and peripheral neuropathy based on the transmitted frequency spectrum and extent of tool acceleration.[59,61] In the usually accepted sense, an ergonomic exposure is something chimeric, because it implies an extrinsic activation and a predictable and graded intrinsic response. While primarily extrinsic factors may predominate in some workplace settings, such as the meatpacking or poultry processing industries, this is not usually the case in the electronic office. Intrinsic elements contribute substantially to tissue response. These human elements of the work process can vary from a mechanical neuromuscular closed loop response to a complex, centrally mediated sequence of subtasks, activities, postures, and patterns that are not appropriately understood as simple responses. The observation that short, small fingers may increase susceptibility to hand pain in electronic keyboard users could simply be considered a pure matter of anthropometry and keyboard design. However, the distinct mechanical advantages of a long finger over a short finger may produce different patterns of adaptation and dynamic movement and distinct patterns of keyboarding movement, some of them potentially injurious.[58] Calling it a short-fingered syndrome is only an introduction to identifying how finger movement is optimized or understanding the learned pattern of integrated finger movement.

PROBLEMS WITH MULTIFACTORIAL DEFINITION

To return to the theme of terminology, given the array of extrinsic and intrinsic components, the variety of work situations in which electronic keyboards are found, and the broad range of medical diagnoses, reliance on a generalizing term has advantages and disadvantages. Accessibility to group analysis requires simplification, but the cost in imprecision may be high.

The usual proposition is that office-related upper extremity disorders result from a complex causal web of work-related factors: biomechanical factors, such as force, static posture, and repetition;[23] psychosocial factors such as job organization and coworker support;[31] and individual susceptibility related to work technique.[25] The default to multiple categories to explain a disease is most often criticized as a refuge for imprecise determination of cause. In fact, the opposite is often true. What have become the most quantitative measurements of keyboard activity—the force and repetition parameters—can be reductionist and simplistic. The measurement of force or output at a given time, determined by a force transducer or indirect measure of output, is a consequence of highly complicated patterns of neuromuscular activation and muscular recruitment and antagonism. Ballistic characteristics are strictly independent variables, indirectly related to the operation of a task, such as reaching the activation threshold of a computer key. The observation that operator-exerted forces on electronic keys significantly exceed necessary key switch force by a large margin that is independent of key resistance[3,25] may obviate a good deal of diversionary research on keyboard design. However, it also underlines the fact that a complex task involves an intricate relationship between the architecture of an external device and internal neuromuscular activity, which may not be easily modeled. Force or output is less a risk factor in the conventional sense than the description of an area ripe with the potential for a misfit between human activity and the device. Pascarelli and Kella observed that a reduced operating force may in fact reflect high levels of intrinsic activity.[58] Electronic microprocessors, which have abbreviated the distance between machine and cognition by replacing a mechanical interface, may also confuse a human design that more slowly coordinates cortical function and mechanical manipulation. In any case, keyboard "force" is less a hard, unitary quantity than a summarization of multiple variables.

A similar issue arises around the terms associated with psychosocial risk factors. The problem again is how to contend with complexity. If the consideration of multiple risk factors means that clinical investigation can proceed by selecting a mood or pain questionnaire, an organizational factor checklist, and placing transducers under a keyboard, the prospects for explicative models will remain dim. Each group of risk factor measurement contains diverse and contradictory premises. It may be better to imagine that there are three independent measurement instruments rather than an integrated approach lying at the intersection of three Boolean circles.

THE USE OF TESTS AND DIFFICULTIES IN ESTABLISHING OBJECTIVE CRITERIA

Clinical medicine proceeds on the basis of objective diagnostic tests or consensual case criteria. Against this standard, many upper extremity disorders associated with the electronic office suffer from lack of definitive objective testing. This is an expectation rather than the exception for soft tissue disorders in general, but it is only part of the reason for diagnostic ambiguity. The problem is that quantitative testing for a syndrome or symptom complex usually provides an abundance of clinical- and test-based information. The selection of a single parameter—a delay in distal median nerve latency, hypesthesia on monofilament testing, or an abnormal Doppler with extreme shoulder contortion—may have no relationship or a tangential relationship to the linking of pathoanatomy and symptoms. Some investigators would base all diagnostic and surgical criteria for carpal tunnel syndrome and release on the electrodiagnostic study to obviate the recognized uncertainties of clinical signs. But decrements in nerve conduction velocity and amplitude may not be reliably associated with seriousness of disease or the need for surgery; the choice of a seemingly high threshold for positive diagnosis may actually mitigate toward overdiagnosis. Nathan presents the problems implicit in basing case definition on an overly sensitive technique. Almost 40% of the tested population met case criteria for CTS, an observation with interesting implications for electrophysiologic measurement but hardly an index of clinical disease, where proportionate normality is expected. The American College of Rheumatology's criteria for fibromyalgia are an example of concurrence on case definition, with no available objective test, but there is such strong disagreement over the diagnosis that the utility of the criteria is problematic. Testing may be important for administrative or medicolegal reasons and may be crucial for longitudinal assessment of populations and clinical management, but there are limits to its usefulness. In some cases, particularly in neurologic testing, the test may yield more information than can be reliably used for case inference.

Another example comes from the study of occupational Raynaud's phenomenon. Cold challenge plethysmography is the test of choice by consensus, experience, and recommendation. However, it diverts attention from symptoms and may not measure cutaneous flow abnormalities. The test has meaning, but it is simply a test and not a representation or recreation of disease paroxysm or process. Hadler's account of a higher prevalence of disabling upper extremity conditions in Denver than in Phoenix telephone operators implicated different, selective, and inappropriate community medical norms as the source of Denver's higher levels of morbidity.[28] However, the issue was a flawed diagnostic and treatment model. If the subject had been tuberculosis screening or sexually transmitted diseases, more intensive organization with lowered surveillance thresholds would also have seen heightened treatment levels and presumably been viewed as beneficial. Treatment patterns have enormous impact on disease recognition but an even more dramatic impact on outcome and efficacy. In our own experience, conservative treatment and workplace modification in the office have been more efficacious in terms of lost-time, morbidity, and cost than surgery. However, invasiveness, with its easily quantifiable upfront costs, has been acceptable to many employers and insurers, and a more aggressive model persists. Although office-related disorders of the upper extremity usually can be addressed by workstation modification and short-term rehabilitative therapy, that is not the prevailing treatment model.

A BROADER SPECTRUM OF EXPOSURE ASSESSMENT: PSYCHOSOCIAL AND ORGANIZATIONAL FACTORS

The body of evidence linking so-called psychosocial, or work organization, factors with musculoskeletal symptoms in the workplace is growing rapidly.[7,10] The term "psychosocial" is a perhaps unfortunate concept, often misused to minimize the physical reality of disease. Additionally, the term sometimes is used to describe the larger, nonwork environment or personal characteristics of workers. This chapter uses the term to refer exclusively to work environmental factors. Much of the research uses the theoretical constructs of demand-control-social support models.[34,37]

NIOSH's newsroom and telecommunications health hazard evaluations implicate a combination of increased job demands and low autonomy in the outbreaks of musculoskeletal disorders at the facilities studied.[8,30] Other studies have consistently found associations between psychological work demands and musculoskeletal disorders in the office. This association is crucial, because so many offices are periodically placed in the throes of yet another technological revolution that is supposed to save time and increase employee productivity. Amick and Damron[2] and other authors demonstrate that the introduction of new office technologies is generally accompanied by a sharp increase in work demands as employees struggle to learn the new technology and work flow while carrying out the existing job tasks. The social system within the workplace often changes dramatically; employees experience losses in contacts with coworkers and supervisors as they spend more time isolated at computer workstations. Many studies have implicated this triad of increased psychological demands, decreased autonomy, and decreased social support in the development of cardiovascular morbidity and mortality.[34,37] More recent work has connected these work organization deficits with musculoskeletal disorders.[32,67] Possible mechanisms through which psychosocial stressors might translate into musculoskeletal disease include increased static muscle contraction, increased blood levels of stress hormones, and even possible disorganization of muscle fiber recruitment and rest cycles.

The effects of increased psychological demands, decreased autonomy, and decreased social supports are especially evident in the misuse of electronic performance monitoring (EPM) in the office environment. Psychosocial deficits in monitored offices have been linked to a wide range of somatic and psychological strain measures, including a number of upper extremity symptoms.[64] In a short experiment, Schleifer et al. found clear EPM-related increases in psychological and physical strain reports over a 3-day period.[62] Even in the absence of EPM, the repetitive data entry tasks studied resulted in increased adverse outcomes. The problems are particularly acute for data entry employees who experience difficulty keeping up with the (externally) established work pace. These and other studies[14] suggest that acute and chronic exposures to the psychosocial stressors associated with computer work in general and monitored computer work in particular may explain a substantial portion of musculoskeletal symptoms in the office environment.

Finally, a full understanding of the causes of upper extremity disorders related to office work requires greater knowledge of company-level structural characteristics and culture. Ivan Most's chapter outlines some organizationally based factors that may affect a call-center employee's decision to report the beginning of musculoskeletal disorders: fear of job loss and reduced opportunities for advancement. Warren's cross-sectional analysis of 528 companies in the Netherlands suggests that a simple hypothesized measure of organizational culture (employer-employee disagreement on risk levels within the company) are strongly associated with musculoskeletal and stress disorders.[67] Similarly, a population-based telephone survey carried out by the University of Connecticut found respondent estimates of organizational support deficits to have stronger associations with musculoskeletal symptom reports than organization measures of demands, low autonomy, and low local social support.[68] In environments such as the office, with less immediately obvious levels of biomechanical stressors, psychosocial and organizational factors may even be more important in the etiology of musculoskeletal disorders than in manufacturing environments.

This chapter has proposed that simple biomechanical stressor characterizations often miss or misrepresent the complex combinations and interactions of neuromuscular and cognitive activities that constitute the highly skilled components of office work. The above research directions strongly suggest that an understanding of the broader combination of biomechanical, psychosocial, and organization-level characteristics is crucial for more effective interventions to reduce office-related upper extremity disorders. To be truly accurate, the overused term "ergonomic exposures" should refer to this greatly expanded range of risk factors rather than only to biomechanical factors.

SUCCESSFUL INTERVENTIONS FOR AN ILL-DEFINED DISEASE

It is important not to underestimate the power of moral persuasion in the introduction of prevention strategies. Many managers and human resources professionals are motivated by a sincere desire to prevent injury to employees and create a healthier and less stressful workplace. But the increased competitive demands of the late 20th century workplace create strong productivity incentives that appear to work against the moral desire to "do the right thing." Thus, it becomes increasingly important to address the true costs to business of an unhealthy workplace. Most larger corporations are now cognizant of factors such as losses in productivity attributable to reduced commitment and quality, increased errors and absenteeism, and elevated recruitment and retraining costs. Office injury-related costs that are borne by individual workers represent economic losses and a wide variety of decrements to the quality of life (see the chapters by Levenstein and by Morse). Although most of these costs are externalized onto the injured worker and, to a degree, onto society, any comprehensive summary of office-related costs should address these issues. But even with these costs not counted, the growing body of collective knowledge in corporate America acknowledges the good business sense of ergonomic prevention efforts.

From the viewpoint of strictly secondary prevention, physical and occupational therapists are developing proven techniques to restore full function to employees with these office-related conditions (see the chapter by Novak and MacKinnon). However, practitioners find that even the best physical medicine procedures are of limited long-term value unless the causative agents in the work environment are simultaneously remediated.

The experience of the University of Connecticut's upper extremity clinic with the home workforce of the Travelers Insurance Company demonstrates the opportunity for a highly effective treatment and intervention strategy, even in the absence of a consensus on the proper term for cases of neck, shoulder, and arm pain that affected a large portion of the office workforce. The program combined an initially entirely empirical application of physical and medical therapeutics with simultaneous workstation changes involving generic alterations in worksite geometry and equipment. The office rapidly receded from being one of the most costly to becoming one of the least costly home offices; surgical rates were reduced by more than tenfold; and overall costs were reduced 78%. This cooperative undertaking earned a designation as "insurance product of the year," a striking accomplishment given the modest theoretic underpinnings of the intervention and the extremely modest, vociferous, and technical controversy over the very definition of these disorders.[35]

Although the joint project focused on medical and engineering aspects of disease, the organizational culture of Travelers is also important. Travelers is a classic Fortune 40 1990s corporation, with a pattern of aggressive acquisition and frequent restructuring, leading to frequent physical changes at the worksite and a shifting middle management structure. This type of button-down hierarchical organization is sometimes characterized as being at high risk for office-related upper extremity disorders. Nevertheless, combined medical and workstation redesign interventions have been effective. In fact, an organizational culture that accepted and promoted the importance of early reporting and workstation remediation is probably one of the primary reasons for the success of the program. Without this underlying organizational commitment, the success of the collaboration would have been far more modest.

Given the emphasis of this chapter on a broader definition of disease and exposure, we will explore examples of interventions directed toward reducing psychosocial and even organizational stressors. Cahill describes a project implemented by the state of New Jersey's child protective agency that was designed to reduce stress-related symptoms through a joint union/management stress committee.[13] The committee used a new computer-based information system to decentralize reporting activities to local offices and improve skill levels and autonomy of office staff.

Simultaneously, office furniture was improved. Over the 6-month follow-up period, employees assessed the psychosocial aspects of the work as being improved. Measures of physical and psychological strain did not change, which was considered a positive finding in light of the tendency of these measures to worsen during times of organizational change.[36] It is also important that this effort had strong union involvement.

The companies with the most successful ergonomics programs seem to accept the maxim that intervention strategies are most effective when introduced using an ergonomics team, with representation from all layers of the organization.[21] It will be interesting to observe over time the subtle results of this approach. By introducing participatory techniques into traditionally hierarchical safety structures, many offices are conducting limited (often unintentional) experiments in work reorganization, thus approaching this chapter's recommendations for combined biomechanical, psychosocial, and organizational prevention strategies. When conducted on a larger scale, these organizational changes do not occur without a temporary cost. Karasek's study of work organization change in Swedish white-collar workers showed that work reorganization often resulted in increased levels of stress and physical symptoms.[36] However, organizational changes characterized by employee input in the change process and increased employee control in the new jobs showed the lowest levels of adverse changes. In addition, the long-term benefits of involving employee and employer in a joint effort to improve the work environment suggest that this temporary cost is more than balanced by the demonstrated reduction in disease and improvement in productivity.[21]

The evidence suggests that upper extremity problems in the office can be relieved relatively easily. If the upper extremity problems of office workers can be so effectively fixed, why should the controversy concerning their very reality exist? One basic explanation is that underlying ideologic and organizational differences are aggravated by semantic imprecision. Another is that acquired terminology shapes and distorts the quality of clinical and epidemiologic investigation. It seems likely that a combination of biomechanical factors, work organization deficits, and underlying organizational factors can account for much of the etiology and exacerbation of office-related upper extremity disorders. However, each piece of this triad includes a complex array of hypotheses and systems of measurement, and the terms themselves are ambiguous. By analogy, the approach of a generation ago that defined coronary heart disease as a consequence of hypertension, cholesterol, and dichotomized personality type has been supplanted by a detailed, mechanistic, and sometimes very different understanding of each of these categories.

Finally, perhaps the primary barrier to implementing the type of participatory intervention found to be most effective in this area is its relative unfamiliarity to a large segment of the industrial and office workplaces in the United States. Unfamiliarity breeds fear. The concepts of information and power sharing that underlie a participatory approach to office work and injury prevention sometimes fly in the face of hierarchical management assumptions. However, we expect that the gains to be realized in terms of improved worker health, reduced costs, and increased productivity will promote the spread of improved work organization in the American workplace.

CONCLUSION

Through much of its history, occupational medicine has approached the exposed and diseased body as a passive medium. When extrinsic exposures in the form of inhalation were associated with pandemics pertinent to specific categories of work that demanded a public health intervention, this mechanistic understanding of disease was satisfactory. Compared to the manufacturing workplace, the evolving electronic workplace—sedentary, more cognitive, and in some respect more standardized in its tasks—often involves a less clear separation of work life from non-work life. While the home office is a more obvious feature of this development, generic therapeutic modifications in work organization are also indices of a blurred margin between job and off-job activities. The tone of common recommendations—hourly rest breaks, home and deskside exercise, attention to stressed muscles and emotions, better posture, weight loss and conditioning—suggests different premises than those that prevail in safety engineering. Likewise, within the office, the separation of physical from mental and even emotional work is increasingly blurred. The interaction between company culture and the biomechanical and psychosocial characteristics of work within the company may be a primary determinant of disease rates in many workplaces. Thus, the epidemic of office-related musculoskeletal disorders pushes theory and practice to widen its scope to become more holistic.

The unsettled discussion over the etiology and even the existence of upper extremity problems in the office is fueled by two very different sources. These are complex dynamic problems that pose great difficulties in the search for underlying mechanisms. Also, the focus on comfort and performance required in the office environment, rather than the elimination of gross external hazards characteristic of manufacturing ergonomics, represents a conceptual shift in the notion of work-related exposure and intervention.

Successful intervention and prevention efforts are currently taking place in offices around the world. Many of the chapters in this volume explore practical approaches to the identification and control of office-related musculoskeletal disorders that are in use by practitioners including physicians, therapists, ergonomists, and organizational consultants. Despite the complexity of disease etiology and the extremely acrimonious and rarefied debate about the existence of these disorders, corporate economic exigencies drive the introduction of empirically based prevention strategies. As often happens in highly politicized scientific controversies, practice currently outruns and will eventually inform theory.

REFERENCES
1. Amadio PC, Russott GM: Evaluation and treatment of hand and wrist disorders in musicians. Hand Clin 6:405–416, 1990.
2. Amick BC, Damron J: A three-year longitudinal assessment of changes in office activities following the introduction of microcomputers into a multinational bank. App Ergon 24:397–404, 1993.
3. Armstrong TJ, Foulke JA, Bernard J, et al: Investigation of applied forces in alphanumeric keyboard work. Am Ind Hyg Assoc J 55:30–35, 1994.
4. Armstrong TJ, Buckle P, Fine LJ, et al: A conceptual model for work-related neck and upper-limb musculoskeletal disorders. Scand J Work Environ Health 19:73–84, 1993.
5. Armstrong TJ, Fine LJ, Goldstein SA, et al: Ergonomics considerations in hand and wrist tendinitis. J Hand Surg 12A(5):830–837, 1987.
6. Bennett JB: Lateral and medial epicondylitis. Hand Clin 10:157–163, 1994.
7. Bernard BP (ed): Musculoskeletal Disorders and Workplace Factors. Cincinnati, National Institute for Occupational Safety and Health, 1997, NIOSH publication 97-141.
8. Barnard B, Sauter S, Petersen M, et al: Health Hazard Evaluation Report. Los Angeles Times, Los Angeles, California. Cincinnati, National Institute for Occupational Safety and Health, 1992, HETA 90-013-2277.
9. Berqvist U, Wolgast E, Nilsson V, Voss M: The influence of VDT work on musculoskeletal disorders. Ergonomics 38:754–762, 1995.
10. Bongers PM, de Winter CR, Kompier MAJ, Hildebrandt VH: Psychosocial factors at work and musculoskeletal disease. Scand J Environ Health 19:297–312, 1993.

11. Brandfonbrener AG: The epidemiology and prevention of hand and wrist injuries in performing artists. Hand Clin 6:365–377, 1990.
12. Bureau of Labor Statistics: Workplace Injuries and Illnesses in 1994. Washington, DC, U.S. Dept. of Labor, 1995, USDL 95-508.
13. Cahill J: Computers and stress reduction in social service workers in New Jersey. Cond Work Digest 11:197–203, 1994.
14. Carayon P: Chronic effect of job control, supervisor social support, and work pressure on office workers stress. In Sauter SL, Murphy LR (eds): Organizational Risk Factors for Job Stress. Washington, DC, American Psychological Association, 1995.
15. Chard MD, Cawston TE, Riley GP, et al: Rotator cuff degeneration and lateral epicondylitis: A comparative histological study. Ann Rheum Dis 53:30–34, 1994.
16. Charness ME, Ross MH, Shefner JM: Ulnar neuropathy and dystonic flexion of the fourth and fifth digits: Clinical correlation in musicians. Muscle Nerve 19:431–437, 1996.
17. Cherniack M: The epidemiology of occupational disorders of the upper extremity. Occup Med State Art Rev 11:487–512, 1996.
18. Cherniack MG: Nonacute musculoskeletal disorders: Then and now. In Erdil M, Dickerson OB (eds): Cumulative Trauma Disorders: Prevention, Evaluation and Treatment. New York, Van Nostrand Reinhold, 1997, pp 25–28.
19. Crowinshield RD, Brand RA, Johnson RC: The effects of walking velocity on hip kinematics and kinetics. Clin Orthop 132:140–144, 1978.
20. Davis RB, Ounpus S, Tsburski D, Gage JR: A gait analysis data collection and reduction technique. Hum Movement Sci 10:575–587, 1991.
21. ErgoWeb, Inc.: Conference Proceedings. Managing Ergonomics in the 1990's. Cincinnati, American Automobile Manufacturers Association and the Center for Office Technology, 1997.
22. Farkkila M, Pyykko I, Jantti V, et al: Forestry workers exposed to vibration: A neurological study. Br J Ind Med 45:188–192, 1988.
23. Faucett J, Rempel D: VDT-related musculoskeletal symptoms: Interactions between work posture and psychosocial work factors. Am J Ind Med 26:597–612, 1994.
24. Ferguson D: The "new" industrial epidemic. Med J Aust 140:318–319, 1984.
25. Feuerstein M, Armstrong T, Pickey P, Lincoln A: Computer keyboard force and upper extremity symptoms. J Occup Environ Med 39:1144–1153, 1997.
26. Fry HJ: Overuse syndrome in musicians: Prevention and management. Lancet 2(8509):728–731, 1986.
27. Gerr F, Letz R, Landrigan PJ: Upper extremity musculoskeletal disorders. Annu Rev Pub Health 12:547–566, 1991.
28. Hadler NM: Arm pain in the workplace; a small area analysis. J Occup Med 34:113–119, 1992.
29. Hadler NM: Clinical perspective: Repetitive upper-extremity motions in the workplace are not hazardous. J Hand Surg 22A:19–29, 1997.
30. Hales T, Sauter S, Petersen M, et al: Health Hazard Evaluation Report. U.S. West Communications. Cincinnati, National Institute for Occupational Safety and Health, 1992, HETA 89-299-2230.
31. Hales TR, Sauter SL, Peterson MR, et al: Musculoskeletal disorders among video display terminal users in a telecommunications company. Ergonomics 37:1603–1621, 1994.
32. Houtman ILD, Bongers PM, Smulders PGW, Kompier MAJ: Psychosocial stressors at work and musculoskeletal problems. Scand J Work Environ Health 20:139–145, 1994.
33. Ireland DCR: Psychological and physical aspects of occupational arm pain. J Hand Surg 13B:5–10, 1988.
34. Johnson JV, Hall EM, Theorell T: Combined effects of job strain and social isolation on cardiovascular disease morbidity and mortality in a random sample of the Swedish male working population. Scand J Work Environ Health 15:271–279, 1989.
35. Kasdan ML: Pathogenesis of cumulative trauma [letter]. J Hand Surg 20:699, 1995.
36. Karasek RA: Lower health risk with increased job control among white collar workers. J Org Behav 11:171–185, 1990.
37. Karasek RA, Theorell T: Healthy Work: Stress, Productivity, and the Reconstruction of Working Life. New York, Basic Books, 1990.
38. Kelsey JL: An epidemiological study of the relationship between occupations and acute herniated lumbar intervertebral discs. Int J Epidemiol 4:197–204, 1975.
39. Keyserling WM: Analysis of manual lifting tasks: A qualitative alternative to the NIOSH work practices guide. Am Ind Hyg Assoc J 50:165–173, 1989.
40. Kissler S, Finholt T: The mystery of RSI. Am Psychol 43:1004–1015, 1988.
41. Koskimies K, Farkkila M, Pyykko I, et al: Carpal tunnel syndrome in vibration disease. Br J Ind Med 47:411–416, 1990.

42. Lederman RJ: Occupational cramp in instrumental musicians. Med Probl Perform Art 3:45–51, 1988.
43. Letz R, Cherniack MG, Gerr R, et al: A cross sectional epidemiological survey of shipyard workers exposed to hand-arm vibration. Br J Med 49:53–62, 1992.
44. Lockwood A: Medical problems of musicians. N Engl J Med 320:221–227, 1989.
45. Lucire Y: Neurosis in the workplace. Med J Aust 145:323–326, 1986.
46. Mandel S: Overuse syndrome in musicians when playing an instrument hurts. Postgrad Med 88:111–114, 1990.
47. Markison RE: Treatment of musical hands: Redesign of the interface. Hand Clin 6:525–544, 1990.
48. Martin BJ, Armstrong TJ, Foulke JA, et al: Keyboard reaction force and finger electromyograms during computer keyboard work. Hum Factors 38:654–664, 1996.
49. MacKinnon SE, Novak CB: Letter to the editor—Reply. J Hand Surg 10A:514, 1994.
50. MacKinnon SE, Novak CB: Clinical perspective: Repetitive strain in the workplace. J Hand Surg 22A:3–18, 1997.
51. McDermott FT: Repetition strain injury: A review of current understanding. Med J Aust 144:196–200, 1986.
52. Masear VR, Hayes JM, Hyde AG: An industrial cause of carpal tunnel syndrome. J Hand Surg 11A:222–227, 1986.
53. Nachemson A: Advances in low-back pain. Clin Orthop 200:266–278, 1985.
54. Nathan PA, Kenniston RC, Meadows KD, Lockwood RS: Therapeutic value of repetitive motion: Work fitness hypothesis, a response to MacKinnon and Novak [letter]. J Hand Surg 20A:513, 1994.
55. Nathan P, Meadows K, Doyle L: Occupation as a risk factor for impaired sensory conduction of the median nerve at the carpal tunnel. J Hand Surg 13B:167–170, 1988.
56. [Reference deleted.]
57. National Institute for Occupational Safety and Health: Health Hazard Evaluation Report. Newsday, Inc., Melville, New York. Cincinnati, National Institute for Occupational Safety and Health, 1990, HETA 89-250-2046.
58. Pascarelli EF, Kella JJ: Soft-tissue injuries related to use of the computer keyboard: A clinical study of 53 severely injured persons. J Occup Med 35:523–532, 1993.
59. Pelmear P, Taraschuk I, Leong D, Wong L: Hand-arm vibration syndrome in foundrymen and hard rock miners. J Low Freq Noise Vibr 5:26–43, 1986.
60. Putz-Anderson V (ed): Cumulative Trauma Disorders: A Manual for Musculoskeletal Diseases of the Upper Limbs. London, Taylor and Francis, 1988.
61. Rawlinson R: Are we assessing hand-arm vibration correctly? J Low Freq Noise Vibr 14:53–60, 1991.
62. Schleifer LM, Galinski TL, Pan CS: Mood disturbance and musculoskeletal discomfort effects of electronic performance monitoring in a VDT data-entry task. In Sauter SL, Murphy LR (eds): Organizational Risk Factors for Job Stress. Washington, DC, American Psychological Association, 1995.
63. Silverstein BA, Fine LJ, Armstrong TJ: Occupational factors and carpal tunnel syndrome. Am J Ind Med 11:343–358, 1987.
64. Smith MJ, Carayon P, Sanders KJ, et al: Employee stress and health complaints in jobs with and without electronic performance monitoring. Appl Ergon 23:17–27, 1992.
65. Spitzer WO, et al: Scientific approach to the assessment and management of activity-related spinal disorders. A monograph for clinicians. Report of the Quebec Task Force on Spinal Disorders. Spine 12:S1–S59, 1987.
66. Reference deleted.
67. Warren N: The organizational and psychosocial bases of cumulative trauma and stress disorders [doctoral dissertation]. Lowell, MA, University of Massachusetts, 1997.
68. Warren N, Dillon C, Morse T, et al: Biomechanical, psychosocial and organizational risk factors for WRMSD; Population-based estimates [manuscript].
69. Weiland AJ: Repetitive strain injuries and cumulative trauma disorders. J Hand Surg 21A:337, 1996.

PAT TITTIRANONDA, PhD
STEPHEN BURASTERO, MD
DAVID REMPEL, MD

RISK FACTORS FOR MUSCULOSKELETAL DISORDERS AMONG COMPUTER USERS

From the Interdisciplinary
  Ergonomics Research Program
Lawrence Livermore National
  Laboratory
Livermore, California (PT, SB)
  and
Division of Occupational and
  Environmental Medicine
Department of Medicine
University of California
San Francisco, California (SB, DR)

Reprint requests to:
Pat Tittiranonda, PhD
Interdisciplinary Ergonomics
  Research Program
Lawrence Livermore National
  Laboratory
7000 East Avenue, L-723
Livermore, CA 94551

The prevalence of musculoskeletal disorders reported in the United States has increased steadily within the past decade, accounting for more than 65% of overall occupational illnesses. Of 308,000 musculoskeletal disorders due to repeated trauma reported in the U.S. workforce in 1995, a total of 92,576 injuries were due to typing or key entry, repetitive tool use, repetitive grasping, pushing, or moving objects other than tools.[15] According to a conservative estimate by the National Institute for Occupational Safety and Health (NIOSH), work-related musculoskeletal disorders cost the U.S. industry more than $13 billion per year.[55]

In the U.S., more than 80 million computers were in use in 1991. By the year 2000, this number is projected to increase to more than 100 million. With such rapid increase in the use of computers both at home and in the workplace, there have been growing concerns over the elevated risks of musculoskeletal disorders.

This chapter reviews the epidemiologic and ergonomic literature that addresses the relationships between occupational factors and upper extremity musculoskeletal disorders (UEMDs) among office workers whose jobs require the operation of video display terminals (VDTs) or alphanumeric keyboards.

MUSCULOSKELETAL DISORDERS

For the purposes of this chapter, musculoskeletal disorders (MSDs) refer to injuries affecting the soft tissues of the neck, shoulder, elbow, hand, wrist, and fingers. These include the nerves (e.g., carpal tunnel syndrome), tendons (e.g., tenosynovitis and epicondylitis), and muscles (e.g., tension neck syndrome).[29,57] The two most frequently studied disorders are carpal tunnel syndrome (CTS) and tendonitis.

Carpal tunnel syndrome (CTS), a condition caused by compression of the median nerve in the carpal tunnel of the wrist, has been reported to be associated with occupational factors such as forceful exertion, repetitive hand motions, awkward postures, mechanical stress, and vibration.[1,6,17–19,21,62–63] Common symptoms are pain, numbness, and tingling in the areas innervated by the median nerve, which include the first three digits of the hand. If left untreated, symptoms can progress to the point at which they interfere with daily activities such as simple manual manipulations, work, or sleep. The diagnosis of CTS is based on the presence of symptoms in the median nerve distribution of the affected hand, physical findings such as Phalen's or Tinel's sign, and positive nerve conduction studies.[29,56] Nonoccupational factors such as systemic diseases (i.e., rheumatoid arthritis, gout, diabetes mellitus, hyperthyroidism), acute wrist trauma,[1] age, female gender,[39,53] use of birth control pills,[58] bilateral oopherectomy,[17] and obesity[49] have been associated with CTS in some studies.

Work-related tendonitis refers to a disorder of the tendons and the tendon sheaths that results from cumulative loading during highly repetitive tasks or forceful tasks involving awkward postures over a prolonged period (Table 1). Patients with tendonitis often complain of localized pain, tenderness, and swelling. Occupational tendonitis can interfere with hand function to the point at which the patient is unable to perform his or her usual work. The diagnosis of tendonitis is based on the presentation of localized pain at the tendon on passive, active, or resisted movement and can be confirmed by aggravation of pain upon palpation. Numerous epidemiologic studies have shown that work-related MSDs are prevalent in industrial settings with similar characteristics, including force, repetition, sustained awkward postures, work and exposure duration, and vibration.

The magnitude of associations between occupational factors and UEMDs varies among studies due to different methods of exposure assessment. Investigators have used job titles, workplace observations of job tasks, checklists, self-reported exposures, hypothesized risk factors associated with certain tasks or occupations, and video and electromyographic analyses of a smaller number of workers within a job to extrapolate exposure status to the study population. The odds ratio for UEMDs found among industrial workers exposed to high force and high repetition compared to those with low force and low repetition varies from 2.6–16.[19,62–63,73]

TABLE 1.   Risk Factors Associated with Musculoskeletal Disorders in Industrial Workers

Risk Factors	References
Forceful exertions	Loupajarvi 1979, Armstrong 1979, Silverstein 1986, Silverstein 1987, Armstrong 1987, Carragee 1988, Chiang 1993
Repetition	Loupajarvi 1979, Kuorinka 1979, Canon 1981, Silverstein 1986, Silverstein 1987, Armstrong 1987, Nathan 1988, Weislander 1989, Barnhart 1991, Chiang 1993
Awkward posture	Loupajarvi 1979, Cannon 1981, Falck 1983, deKrom 1990, Barnhart 1991, Marras 1993
Mechanical stress	Armstrong 1986, Tichauer 1966
Vibration	Cannon 1981, Weislander 1989

Jobs that involve repetitive or static awkward deviations (i.e., wrist flexion, extension, ulnar or radial deviations) have demonstrated odds ratios from 4.9–8.1.[6,21,43,46] Duration of work involving flexed and extended wrists and cumulative exposure to vibration have shown an exposure-effect relationship.[17,21] Exposure to vibration has shown odds ratios greater than 4.[17,73] Studies on the effects of work-related factors such as forcefulness, repetitive movements, and vibration on UEMDs in industrial settings have been consistent in the epidemiologic literature.[55]

STUDIES OF MUSCULOSKELETAL DISORDERS AMONG COMPUTER USERS

Some ergonomic risk factors associated with MSDs in industrial settings are also present in the operation of VDTs and alphanumeric keyboards, including repetitive motion (20,000–200,000 keystrokes per day);[5] sustained static neck, shoulder, and hand postures;[27,36] and force.[5] Epidemiologic studies evaluating UEMDs have been conducted among various jobs requiring the use of keyboards (i.e., telegraphists, accounting machine operators, programmers, newspaper employees, and directory assistant operators). Researchers have evaluated the relationship of physical and work organizational factors of computer work to symptoms of UEMDs. Most studies are cross-sectional and are based on self-reported health measures. As is the case for epidemiologic studies conducted on industrial populations, workplace factors are frequently assessed by questionnaires, and few studies have used job sampling methods, video analyses, or measurements of work posture and workstations to characterize exposure related to VDT use. Criteria for case definitions also differ between studies, limiting possible comparisons. Some studies have based their case definitions on self-reported symptoms alone, and others define MSD cases by both symptoms and clinical findings. A series of studies conducted by NIOSH have used standardized physical examinations and case definitions and, thus, can be directly compared.[7,16,34]

In studies examining the relationships between occupational stress and UEMDs, various psychosocial measures have been used. Prevalidated, factor-analyzed instruments were often used to assess psychosocial aspects of the work environment in NIOSH's studies. Several researchers have adopted the Karasek's Job Content Instrument to measure stress.[38] The Karasek Index has been standardized and extensively used to study the effects of stress on heart disease.

Studies also have differed in their approach to statistical analyses. Early studies used univariate statistics and often neglected the effects of multivariate relationships and confounding variables. Recent studies have used multivariate statistical techniques to explore the associations and interactions of one or more independent variables in MSDs. A review of these studies follows.

In 1971, occupational cramps and myalgia were reported among Australian telegraphists who used conventional QWERTY electric alphanumeric keyboards.[26] Medical interviews and physical examinations of 516 male telegraphists from several Australian public service organizations were carried out from 1958–1963. A total of 14% of the subjects were diagnosed with occupational cramp (defined as incoordination, stiffness, spasm, weakness, tremor, and pain or disturbance of sensation in the operating limb), and 5% were diagnosed with occupational myalgia (defined as complaint of aches and pain in the neck, shoulder, arm, forearm, or wrist after 30 minutes of working at their job). The authors observed that occurrence of these symptoms may be related to "adverse" work postures during keyboard use and attributed these postures to keyboard design flaws. To confirm their hypothesis, the authors carried out a nested case-control study to examine the relationship between keyboard operating postures and symptoms (see page 31).

In a cross-sectional study, Maeda et al. used a questionnaire and body diagrams to determine the prevalence of physical discomfort among accounting machine operators in Japan.[44] A total of 110 female accounting machine operators, who were required to enter data with their right hand into a numeric keyboard, were compared to 57 saleswomen who had no exposure to a cash register or other machines. Subjects rated symptoms of tiredness, pain, and numbness for each part of their body, and certain aspects of their workstations were measured. The prevalence of pain and tiredness in the right and left hand were significantly higher (Mann-Whitney U tests, $p < 0.01$) among the accounting machine operators than the saleswomen. For the accounting machine operators, the mean table and keyboard heights were reported to be too high. For both groups, awkward work postures were qualitatively described.

Hunting et al. published a series of studies in 1981–1985.[31,37] The first study of the series evaluated the association between awkward typing postures and physical discomfort with the use of a conventional keyboard. In this study, the authors[37] used the same questionnaire as Maeda et al.[44] in evaluating full-time typists versus traditional office workers who used a keyboard occasionally (controls). Medical examinations were conducted, a survey of work satisfaction was administered, and work postures were measured. The authors found an elevated incidence of self-reported pain in the upper extremities and positive medical findings among the 240 keyboard/typewriter users compared to the 55 controls. More than 10% of the computer user group and 0–2% of the controls reported daily pain for the neck, shoulder, upper extremity, and lumbar regions. Positive medical findings of painful pressure points at the muscles and tendons and forearm pain during isometric contraction were three times higher for the keyboard operator group and were associated with awkward body postures.

In 1982, Bell Telephone Laboratories carried out a questionnaire-based, cross-sectional survey of telephone operators.[68] The growing reports of computer-related MSDs had prompted this investigation because more than 130,000 computers were in use in the Bell System during that time. Participants included 145 directory assistance operators who used computers and 105 controls who carried out a similar task using a printed document. Of those solicited, 95% of the paper operators and 76% of the computer operators volunteered. Participants were selected randomly from the volunteers and completed a self-administered checklist to assess symptoms and a questionnaire regarding job satisfaction and security. Results showed that, within the previous month, the proportion of the computer users who reported discomfort was not significantly higher than the control group, except for neck discomfort ($\chi^2 = 5.18$, $p < 0.05$) and mean symptom index (6.7 vs. 5.4, $p < 0.005$). After controlling for age, however, no significant association was detected. Starr and colleagues explained that the prevalence of discomfort among the controls was underestimated due to a higher distribution of older workers who reported fewer complaints. They concluded that "replacing paper documents with computers need not adversely affect the comfort and morale of office workers."

In 1984, NIOSH conducted a health hazard evaluation of clerical workers at a police department.[60] An initial cross-sectional survey of 33 clerk/typists showed that six of 10 police transcribers but one of 22 staff members from other departments reported medical diagnoses of CTS or tendonitis. The diagnoses were confirmed by medical records or physicians (odds ratio [OR] = 31.5, $p < 0.001$). Interestingly, patients with CTS or tendonitis reported a shorter term of employment than patients without CTS or tendonitis (5.3 years ± 4.3 vs. 11.8 years ± 8.9, respectively). A potential survivor bias (i.e., some transcribers may have changed jobs because of MSD problems) may have caused the odds ratio to be underestimated.

In 1989, NIOSH conducted a cross-sectional study of newspaper employees at Newsday.[16] The authors used a questionnaire to measure exposures and symptoms. Hand and body diagrams were used to determine the areas of pain or discomfort, and the case definitions for MSDs were based on medical history alone. Criteria for work-related MSDs, which were also used in subsequent NIOSH studies, are as follows:

1. Pain, aching, stiffness, burning, tingling or numbness
2. Symptoms must occur within the past year and last for ≥ 1 week or occur at least once/month
3. No previous accident or acute injury to the joints within the past year
4. Symptoms must occur on the current job

Based on the questionnaire, 40% of the 836 participants reported symptoms consistent with UEMDs: hand/wrist symptoms (23%), neck (17%), elbow/forearm (13%), and shoulder (11%). Logistic regression analyses indicated that after controlling for speed, reporters had significantly higher odds of developing hand/wrist (OR = 2.4, 95% confidence interval [CI] = 1.6–3.4) and elbow/forearm symptoms (OR = 2.5, 95% CI = 1.5–4.0). Symptoms of the hand/wrist, elbow/forearm, shoulder, and neck were all reported to be associated with typing on computer keyboards.

In 1992, Bernard et al. from NIOSH performed a cross-sectional study of 973 newspaper employees at the *Los Angeles Times* in response to a health hazard evaluation request.[7,8] Their questionnaires and case definition were similar to those used in the 1989 study. Results showed that 41% (395/973) of the participants reported significant work-related UEMDs within the past year, including neck symptoms (26%), hand/wrist (22%), shoulder (17%), and elbow symptoms (10%). The prevalence of disorders of the hand and wrist were consistent with findings of other studies of newspaper employees, which have reported prevalences of 17–26%.[14,50,51,56] In addition, the odds for having hand and wrist symptoms were reported to increase in a dose-response manner; more than a twofold risk was observed among those who typed 6–8 hours compared to those who spent 0–2 hours typing (OR = 2.5, 95% CI = 1.6–3.9). Overall, potential selection bias was minimized because the response rate was high (95%), and survivor bias was not considered problematic because few employees had terminated their employment during the previous year.

Another cross-sectional study by NIOSH of 533 computer users at a telecommunications company in the Midwest showed that 22% of the employees met the case definition of work-related UEMDs based on symptom questionnaires and physical examinations.[34–35] The hand and wrist area was the most affected (12%), followed by the neck (9%), elbow (7%), and shoulder area (6%). According to the authors, the prevalence rates were half those previously reported among newspaper employees. This drop was due to the use of a more restrictive case definition, which included positive medical examination findings in addition to the symptom questionnaires. Strengths and limitations similar to previous NIOSH studies were addressed. The results of this study, however, conflict with the previous study of directory assistance operators at Bell System, conducted approximately 10 years earlier.[68] Starr et al. failed to find a significant risk associated with computer use.[68] The small sample size in Starr's study (n = 145) may have been inadequate to detect real differences between groups. In addition, use of a physical discomfort checklist rather than body diagrams may not have been as specific in detecting MSD. The lower response rate (76% among the computer users) may have led to selection and survivor biases.

Faucett and Rempel[24] used a questionnaire to investigate the interrelationship between work posture, job characteristics, and interpersonal relationships and the severity of MSD symptoms among 150 newspaper employees at the *San Francisco Chronicle*.[24] The sample size was smaller than in previous NIOSH studies, and the study included only employees from the editorial department. The *Los Angeles Times* evaluation consisted of employees from four departments: editorial, finance, circulation, and classified.[7-8] The case criteria were different. Hand and body diagrams were incorporated into the questionnaire, and MSD was defined by pain, numbness, or stiffness of at least 2 on the 10-point severity scale. The authors found that 23% of the respondents reported pain in the upper extremity regions in the preceding week and 19% had symptoms consistent with the case definition for a potential UEMD. The prevalence rate of 38% for MSDs was lower than the figure reported by NIOSH.[7] Such discrepancy may be explained by the fact that symptoms were based on the preceding week instead of the previous year, as used in NIOSH studies. Additional analyses of risk factors for potential MSDs have demonstrated that the risk of an upper extremity disorder increased 1.49 times with increasing daily hours of computer use (95% CI = 1.10–2.02). Other aspects of this analysis are described in the next section.

The only prospective study of MSDs among computer users was conducted in 1981–1987 in Sweden.[9-11] Of the 535 office workers participating in 1981, 353 (66%) remained in the study in 1987. Musculoskeletal discomfort was assessed using the Nordic questionnaire.[41] To assess a potential survivor bias, questionnaires were sent to the subjects who dropped out during the study. The questionnaire asked if specific health problems or computer work had "strongly contributed" to the subject's decision to leave the job. Survivor bias, calculated based on this questionnaire, was found to potentially lead to an underestimation of the risk ratios by 20% for the back and 40% for the hand/wrist. Despite such risk ratio underestimation, the authors found that computer users of at least 6 years are 2.6 times more likely to develop hand and wrist symptoms than noncomputer users (95% CI = 0.7–9.38).

In 1990, Marcus and Gerr[45] conducted a questionnaire-based cross-sectional study of female office workers at three companies in the New York City metropolitan area. Of 645 women who were invited to participate, 467 (70%) completed the questionnaires. The authors derived their symptom questionnaire, which included hand and body diagrams, from what was previously used in NIOSH studies.[7,16,34] A similar case definition was used, but medical examinations were not carried out. Similar to other epidemiologic studies, they found an elevated incidence of upper extremity symptoms among female office workers who reported "ever using a VDT." A total of 63% reported symptoms in the neck or shoulder region, and 34% reported arm or hand symptoms. In addition, workers who reported ever using a computer were more likely than the noncomputer users to report hand/arm symptoms (OR = 3.87, 95% CI = 1.24–12.02). A higher prevalence of both hand/arm and neck/shoulder symptoms was also found among the group who at one point used a computer (40–60% vs. 30% among nonusers). Based on these findings, the authors suggested that the effect of survivor bias may exist and may reduce reported association between computer use and MSDs and distort the results of some cross-sectional studies.

All but one[68] of the studies reviewed in this chapter showed evidence of elevated MSD risks associated with computer or keyboard use (Table 2). The prevalences of MSDs among computer users was higher than controls. Keyboard-related MSDs prevalences varied between 9–50% compared to 4.5–17% among the reference

TABLE 2. Epidemiologic Studies of Work-Related Musculoskeletal Disorders in Office Settings

References	Study Design	Study Population	Exposure Measures	Outcome Measures	Relative Risks	95% CI	Exposed Prevalence/ Incidence	Referent Prevalence/ Incidence
Ferguson & Duncan 1974[27]	Case-Control	90 telegraphists with occupational cramps & myalgia (identified from previous study, Ferguson, 1972) vs. 45 nonsymptomatic telegraphists of similar age, gender, & job tasks	Awkward postures, i.e., shoulder abduction, wrist extension, ulnar deviation among 29 cases & 45 controls were examined	Diagnosis made by a physiotherapist. "Occupational cramps: "functional incoordination of an accustomed repetitive skill, akin to a habit spasm." Occupational myalgia: "current muscle-aching associated with continued repetitive tasks."	Shoulder abduction Wrist extension Ulnar deviation	10.9 4.2 3.5		
Maeda et al. 1980[44]	Cross-Sectional	119 accounting machine operators vs. 57 sales women in a department store	Static posture measurements 1) forward neck flexion 2) use of right hand to operate numeric keyboard 3) repetition—8,000–12,000 strokes/hr 4) work hours—44 hours/week Saleswomen selling goods without operating cash registers (walking, standing, bending down)	Questionnaire was used to rate symptoms of stiffness, tiredness & pain for each body part	Arm pain "machine operator" Hand pain "machine operator"	3.4 2.0	45% 49%	17% 10%
Hunting et al. 1980[36]	Case-Control	Subset of Maeda's 57 accounting machine operators	Static postures: head and trunk inclinations, left/right arm abduction, extension and ulnar deviation	Refer to Maeda et al. 1980	Hand pain	5.7	ulnar deviation >20° 70%	<9° 40%
Hunting et al. 1981[37]	Cross-Sectional	162 VDT operators (data entry & conversational terminals, 105 females) operators vs. 55 traditional office workers (33 females)	Keying 12,000–17,000 strokes/hr vs. occasional keyboard use with diverse movement among the traditional office workers	Questionnaire (Maeda et al. 1980) and medical exams-palpation of painful pressure points in shoulders, arms, hands and painful symptoms in isometric contraction of the forearms	Arm/Elbow data entry conversational Ulnar deviation data entry conversational	8.0 2.8 >20° 6.3 8.8	Painful isometric contraction 21%	6%

Table continued on next page.

TABLE 2. Epidemiologic Studies of Work-Related Musculoskeletal Disorders in Office Settings (Cont.)

References	Study Design	Study Population	Exposure Measures	Outcome Measures	Relative Risks	95% CI	Exposed Prevalence/ Incidence	Referent Prevalence/ Incidence
Starr et al. 1982[08]	Cross-Sectional	Director assistants—250 VDT users from 7 offices vs. 105 non-VDT users from 3 offices	Use of VDT vs. printed paper to obtain directory listings		wrist elbow upper arm	0.67 — 0.79 — 1.10 —	10% 9% 14%	14% 11% 13%
Knave et al. 1985[40]	Cross-Sectional	400 VDT operators from an insurance airline, post office & newspaper companies who worked > 5 hrs/day vs. workers performing similar tasks, but did not use VDT	Self-reported VDT work (yrs and hrs/wk), hrs of VDT work—infrared transmitter attached to spectacles used to measure time spent looking at VDT screen (surrogate measure of VDT hours)	Subjective reporting of symptoms & discomfort. Discomfort index constructed for musculoskeletal complaints	Total daily work hrs greater among those with musculoskeletal discomfort			
Seligman et al. 1984[40]	Case-Control	10 police transcribers compared to 23 other clerks and typists	Ergonomic assessments based on analysis of wrist ulnar/radial deviations; keying and keystrokes/second were also measured	Medical reports of numbness or pain in the median nerve distribution of the hand, positive Tinel's or Phalen's tests or EMG/NCV	Wrist extension greater among cases than controls		20% 50%	4.5% 4.5%
Nathan et al. 1988[48]	Cross-Sectional	22 keyboard operators (> 4hr/day) vs. 147 administrative/clerical staff (< 4hr/day of keyboard use)	Job classification	Sensory latencies of the median nerve maximum latency difference ≥ 0.4 ms was considered abnormal	2.75		Bilateral median nerve slowing 18%	8%
Burt et al. 1990[16]	Cross-Sectional	834 newspaper employees from 4 buildings	% time spent typing, typing speed, reporter, break from workstation, keying outside of work, all based on self reports	Questionnaire-based case definition; (1) pain, numbness, stiffness, burning, within preceding year in shoulder, elbow, hand & wrist (2) no previous accidents or injuries (3) symptoms began on current job (4) symptoms lasted > 1 week or at least > 1 month	Reporter 2.5 Typing speed slow 0.9 moderate 1.3 fast 2.5	1.6–3.4 0.3–2.3 0.6–3.1 1.6–3.4	Period Prevalence Rate hand/wrist 22%	

Table continued on next page.

TABLE 2. Epidemiologic Studies of Work-Related Musculoskeletal Disorders in Office Settings (Cont.)

References	Study Design	Study Population	Exposure Measures	Outcome Measures	Relative Risks	95% CI	Exposed Prevalence/ Incidence	Referent Prevalence/ Incidence
Bernard et al. 1993[7]	Cross-Sectional	973 newspaper employees from accounting, editorial, classified & circulation departments (396 females & 577 males)	Self reported typing hrs/day, hrs on deadline/wk, time spent on work variance, # years employed	Refer to Burt et al. 1990 In addition, the intensity of symptom must be "moderate" on the intensity	hrs. typing/day (6–8 vs. 0–2 hrs) 2.5; deadline hrs/wk (30–39 vs. 0–10 hrs) 1.6; typing hours 0–<2 1.0, 2–<4 1.0, 4–<6 1.3, 6–<8 2.1, ≥8 3.3	1.6–3.9; 1.2–2.3; 0.6–1.8, 0.8–2.2, 1.3–3.6, 1.2–8.9	Period Prevalence Rate hand/wrist 22%	
Faucett & Rempel 1994[24]	Cross-Sectional	150 VDT operators from an editorial department of a newspaper company	Observations on work postures, knee & leg contact with keyboard relative to elbow height, relative seat-back height, self-measures of psychosocial work factors on subset of 70 workers	Self-administered questionnaire using body diagram. Case definition (1) pain, numbness or stiffness of at least 2 on severity scale and ≥ 2 days in past week (2) symptoms improved on days off work	Greater hrs of VDT use 1.49	1.1–2.02	Period Prevalence Rate > 9% met criteria for potential UEMD –14% upper body disorders	

Table continued on next page.

TABLE 2. Epidemiologic Studies of Work-Related Musculoskeletal Disorders in Office Settings (Cont.)

References	Study Design	Study Population	Exposure Measures	Outcome Measures	Relative Risks	95% CI	Exposed Prevalence/ Incidence	Referent Prevalence/ Incidence
Bergqvist et al. 1995[10]	Cross-Sectional	260 computer workers	Workplace investigation was conducted to assess static work postures, use of arm support, nonneutral postures, repeated movement, leg space, relative keyboard and elbow height	Musculoskeletal discomfort obtained from a Nordic questionnaire. Physical exams also conducted. Case definitions: (1) aches, stiffness, tiredness, numbness in the neck, shoulder, elbows and hands for at least 1 week or >20 times during the previous year (2) diabetes, inflammatory diseases & trauma were excluded	**Arm/hand discomfort** nonneutral hand posture 3.8 low keyboard 2 **Hand Disorders** 1) limited break 2.7 2) nonuse of arm support 2.7 3) interaction between 1 and 2 10.1	1.0–15.0 0.9–4.5 0.8–9.1 0.9–8.3 2.4–43.2	Period Prevalence Rate hand/arm sx 30% hand/arm disorders 9%	
Bergqvist et al. 1995[11]	Prospective	322 office workers	Self-reports of VDT use, categorized into data entry or interactive VDT users. Assessments of ergonomic factors were carried out in the same way as Bergqvist 1995[47]	Neck/shoulder, lower back and arm/hand discomforts in the last 12 months were determined by the Nordic questionnaire. Clinical exams include diagnosis of tension neck syndrome, cervical syndrome and any shoulder and arm/hand diagnoses	**Arm/hand Discomfort** 2 VDT work > 5 py 1.4 VDT work 5–20 hr/wk 1.6 VDT work ≥ 20 hr/wk 1.8 **Hand Disorders** limited break and nonuse of lower arm support in those worked ≥ 20 hr/wk 4.6	0.7–2.8 0.8–4.5 0.8–3.9 1.2–17.9	hand/arm sx 29% hand/arm disorders 9%	

Table continued on next page.

TABLE 2. Epidemiologic Studies of Work-Related Musculoskeletal Disorders in Office Settings (Cont.)

References	Study Design	Study Population	Exposure Measures	Outcome Measures	Relative Risks	95% CI	Exposed Prevalence/ Incidence	Referent Prevalence/ Incidence
Marcus & Gerr 1996[45]	Cross Sectional	409 female office workers, age ≤ 40 yrs from three companies	Self assessment of years of VDT use, current VDT use (hr/wk), exercise frequency, job stress & social support	Case definitions derived from NIOSH (Burt et al. 1990 & Bernard et al. 1993) Case definition for arm/hand symptoms: pain or sorenes in the fingers, hands, wrists, forearms or, numbness or tingling of the fingers ≥ once per week or at least of moderate intensity during the previous month	VDT use (yrs) 0 yr 1.0 < 3 yrs 1.9 4–6 yrs 1.9 > 6 yrs 3.9	— 0.7–5.2 0.7–5.3 1.2–12.0	Period Prevalence Rate hand/arm symptoms 34.2%	

VDT = video display terminal; EMG = electromyography; NCV = nerve conduction velocity

groups who were exposed to low or no keyboard work. Among the groups of computer users, the prevalence rate based on symptom and/or physical examination findings for the neck and shoulder ranged from 6–49% and from 9–50% for the hand, wrist, and elbow (see Table 2). Overall, the risk for neck/shoulder disorders was 0.5–9.9, and the risk for hand, wrist, and elbow disorders ranged from 0.7–10.1 for computer users compared to controls. In a review of epidemiologic studies of MSDs in computer keyboard use by Punnett,[54] external comparisons were made between a series of cross-sectional studies conducted by NIOSH.[7–8,16,34–35] and a study of industrial workers by Silverstein et al.[62–63] After gender adjustment, the prevalences of hand and wrist symptoms and disorders were approximately two to eight times higher than the rates reported for low-force and low-repetition industrial jobs and were the same or higher than the rates for high-repetition and low-force industrial jobs.

Similar to the industrial populations, excess risks of developing UEMDs have been observed for work tasks that involve repetitiveness. Repetitive keying from 8,000–12,000 strokes per hour was found to be associated with increased risks of arm, hand, and elbow pain compared to job tasks involving walking, standing, or bending.[36,44] In three cross-sectional studies, intensity (e.g., typing speed) and duration of computer use (e.g., daily and weekly typing hours and years of computer use) showed an exposure-effect relationship (see Table 2).[7–8,16,45] Activities involving nonneutral wrist postures, which were associated with CTS and tendonitis in industrial populations, were also reported among office workers. Typing in wrist extension or ulnar deviation showed an increased MSD risk that ranged from 3.8–8.8 (see Table 2).[11,27,36,60]

RISK FACTORS ASSOCIATED WITH MUSCULOSKELETAL DISORDERS DURING COMPUTER WORK

Specific risk factors that may be associated with computer work include repetitive and sustained exertions, forceful exertions, awkward postures, and localized mechanical stresses. Although the pathophysiologic mechanisms linking keyboard use to MSDs are not fully established, the conceptual model as proposed by Armstrong et al. can be applied.[4] When operating a keyboard, repetitive key entry (50,000–200,000 keystrokes per day) may cause irritation to the membranes surrounding the extensor tendons (synovial sheaths) or the tendons themselves. Moving the fingers repetitively while the wrist is flexed, extended, or ulnar-deviated can cause the flexor tendons to move past and against the walls of the carpal tunnel.[2] Such movements can create contract forces between the tendons and the adjacent walls and in turn can cause inflammation and swelling of the tendons and synovial membranes. Repetitive loading over time increases the carpal canal pressure and may cause median nerve compression. Repetitive finger and wrist movements also can affect the flexor and extensor muscles of the forearms. Mechanical and physiologic changes such as muscle tissue deformation, depletion of nutrients and blood flow, and accumulation of metabolites can lead to fatigue and discomfort. When muscle fatigue occurs daily without sufficient recovery, muscle injuries may result. Additionally, when using the keyboard, contact forces that can occur when the wrist is pressed against the sharp edge of the table or hard surface can cause direct compression to the underlying tendons and nerves. Finger forces applied during typing may create additional stresses to the tendons. Loading of the flexor tendons causes an increase in carpal tunnel pressure[65] and may contribute to the development of MSDs. Physical and personal risk factors reported to be associated with keyboard-related UEMDs are described below.

Physical Risk Factors

TYPING DURATION

Among the studies conducted on newspaper employees, Burt et al. found an increased risk of elbow/forearm MSD symptoms with an increasing percentage of the time spent typing on a computer keyboard.[16] Employees who spent 80–100% of their time typing had an odds ratio of 2.8 (95% CI = 1.4–5.7) compared to those who spent 19% or less of their time typing. A follow-up study conducted on the same population found subjects with hand/wrist symptoms to report a significantly greater percentage of their time keying (51.1%) than asymptomatic subjects (44.6%) (p < 0.03).[64]

Bernard et al. reported reported results that supported an exposure-response relationship between daily typing hours and MSD of the hand and wrist.[7,8] In comparison to the reference group (0–2 hours of typing per day), newspaper employees who reported typing 6–8 hours per day were 2.1 times more likely to have hand/wrist disorders (95% CI = 1.3–3.6), and the odds increased to 3.3 (95% CI = 1.2–8.9) if they reported typing more than 8 hours per day. The authors were also able to verify through job sampling that 36 randomly selected subjects with hand/wrist symptoms spent significantly more time typing (2.5 hours ± 1.9) than the 40 controls (1.9 hours ± 0.9) (t test, p < 0.02). Work sampling results suggested that although self-reported hours of typing were overestimated when compared with direct observation, symptomatic subjects did not overestimate the hours spent typing in comparison to the controls.

In another cross-sectional study of newspaper reporters and editors, Faucett and Rempel found an increased risk of having a potential UEMD with a greater number of self-reported daily hours of VDT use (OR = 1.49, 95% CI = 1.1–2.0).[24]

In a cross-sectional investigation of 565 Stockholm office workers conducted in 1981, a more objective technique of assessing work hours was carried out on a subgroup of 132 individuals.[40] A gaze direction instrument was used to determine the amount of time subjects spent looking at a VDT (a surrogate measure for VDT work hours). During the course of a work day, a special infrared receiver was placed on top of the VDT to detect signals from the transmitter that was attached to the subjects' normal or hollow spectacles. The authors found that subjects who experienced MSDs worked significantly longer (6.2 hours) than asymptomatic subjects (5.4 hours) (p < 0.05).

In a follow-up, cross-sectional study of the same cohort in 1987, Bergqvist et al. defined VDT use by the total cumulative hours of VDT work reported on the questionnaires in 1981 and again in 1987.[10] In this study, users (> 20 hours of VDT use per week) and nonusers (< 5 hours of VDT use per week) were compared. VDT users were found to exhibit an increased odds ratio of hand/arm (OR = 4.6, 95% CI = 1.2–17.9) and tension neck syndrome diagnoses (OR = 6.9, 95% CI = 1.1–42.1) when external workplace factors were controlled for.

Marcus and Gerr reported a complex relationship between self-reported computer use and MSD symptoms.[45] In their initial analyses, they found no association between duration of computer use (hours per week or years of computer use) and MSD reporting. In fact, subjects who reported current computer use (> 5 hours per week) were less likely than the noncurrent computer users to report hand/arm symptoms. Interestingly, when computer use was redefined to include former and current users, subjects who reported ever using a computer for more than 6 years were more likely than the non-VDT users to report hand/arm symptoms (OR = 3.87, 95% CI = 1.24–12.02). A higher prevalence of both hand/arm and neck/shoulder symptoms were also found among the group that at one point used a computer (40–60% vs. 30% among nonusers). Within this group, former users reported a higher prevalence of MSD symptoms than the current users (i.e., 60% of former users of > 6 years vs. 43% of current users of the same duration). Based on these findings, the authors suggested that survivor bias may exist and may lead to the lack of an association between computer use and the reporting of MSDs in some studies. For example, Sauter et al. reported that hours using a computer, as categorized in 10-hour increments, did not have an influence on physical discomfort in a study of 539 data entry computer users.[24] Hales and Sauter found an inverse association between hours spent at a computer per day and potential hand/wrist symptoms among 511 telecommunications employees ($R^2 = 0.02$, $p < 0.05$).[35] Because selection criteria required the employees to use a computer at least 6 hours per day, the mean number of computer hours was 7.3 ± 0.95. The authors concluded that due to the lack of variation in hours of computer use per day, the association between computer use and MSDs could not be accurately evaluated. "Self-selection bias" may occur when asymptomatic employees volunteer for overtime work or symptomatic workers do not volunteer or are not permitted by their supervisors to work overtime. In summary, computer use may lead to MSD symptoms, but users who experience symptoms are likely to reduce their use of computers or may no longer be working when epidemiologic studies are being carried out.

According to the literature, increased typing duration, measured by a subjective estimation of typing (hours/day) or cumulative VDT use (years) is strongly associated with increased MSD risks. The risks of arm, hand, and wrist disorders for keyboard or VDT use of more than 4 hours per day ranged from 1.5–4.6. An elevated risk of 3.9 was also reported for cumulative exposure to VDT (> 6 years) compared to non-VDT users. MSDs may result from daily exposure of tissues to exertions of the muscles, tendons, and nerves during repetitive keying. Chronic impairment may develop when repair capacity is reduced or when repair cannot take place as quickly as damage occurs.

Typing Speed

Burt et al. and Silverstein et al. found that increased risks of hand/wrist and shoulder symptoms were associated with self-reported typing speed.[16,64] For hand/wrist symptoms, the odds ratios for slow, moderate, and fast typists were 0.9 (95% CI = 0.3–2.3), 1.3 (95% CI = 0.6–3.1) and 2.5 (95% CI = 1.0–5.6), respectively.

In a laboratory-based study, Gerard et al. examined the effects of typing speed on muscle activity as well as the reporting of perceived discomfort and exertion among 18 subjects.[28] Typing speeds under three conditions (self-paced, 50% maximum typing speed, and 100% maximum typing speed) were controlled by the scrolling speed of the text. The authors found that more muscle activity and fatigue occurred when typing at the faster speeds. There were also significant increases in perceived localized muscle fatigue ($p < 0.01$ or greater) when typing at maximum speed.

Based on the conceptual model of MSD pathogenesis, faster typists may be at a higher risk due to the greater amount of repetitive keying per day with less recovery time between successive exertions. Repetitive and prolonged exertions of the muscles and tendons with inadequate recovery time can lead to tendon deformation and energy depletion in the muscles, which can in turn lead to fatigue and pain.

Work-Rest Cycles

In a comparative study of 260 VDT users (> 20 hours per week) and 60 nonusers (< 5 hours per week), Bergqvist et al. found that users were 4.6 times more likely than nonusers (95% CI = 1.2–17.9) to have arm/hand disorders diagnoses if they did not have an opportunity for limited rest breaks and at the same time did not use lower arm support.[10]

In a case study of 85 VDT operators, paid exercise breaks (two 5-minute sessions of arm, neck, back, and leg stretching and manipulation per day) in addition to regular rest breaks increased productivity (defined as average number of items processed per operator) by 25% compared to the previous year.[72] Following the introduction of the exercise break program, the number of MSD-related workers' compensation claims fell. The authors concluded that mini-breaks, when interspersed throughout the workday, are effective in preventing the gradual build-up of muscular strains that may lead to physical discomfort.

Hagberg and Sudelin[33] measured changes in activity of the trapezius muscles and subjective discomfort level among six female VDT word processors while they engaged in (1) 5 hours of continuous work with regular lunch and coffee breaks, (2) 3 hours of continuous work with coffee breaks, and (3) 3 hours of work with 10 short pauses every hour. Short pauses were administered by playing "soft music" for 15 seconds, every sixth minute, to remind each subject to take breaks. The authors reported a significant decrease in the discomfort ratings for all body regions (eyes, neck, shoulders, hands, elbows and back) (p < 0.01, Mann Whitney U) for the work period in which short pauses were introduced. However, the authors were unable to demonstrate the difference in muscular activities between the three work conditions, possibly due to a small sample size.

Evidence regarding the role of the work-rest cycle during keyboard work in the development of MSDs has been limited. It is biologically plausible that exceeding a certain load-rest level may cause irreversible damage to the tendons. Goldstein et al. have demonstrated that tendon elongation, a response to tensile loads, is irreversible when insufficient time is given between successive loads.[30]

NONNEUTRAL JOINT POSTURES

Duncan and Ferguson conducted a follow-up nested case-control study of 90 male teleprinters with a confirmed medical diagnosis of cramp and myalgia and 45 controls.[22] Based on qualitative observations, a significantly greater percentage of cases than controls were found to assume shoulder abduction, defined as "when the elbow was carried out appreciably to the side from the normal vertical hang of the upper arm (58% cases vs. 12% controls, χ^2, p < 0.001); ulnar deviation, defined as "when the hand was held definitely turned out at the wrist as viewed in the prone operating posture of the hand" (70% cases vs. 39% controls, p < 0.001); and wrist extension, defined as "bending back up (of the wrist) (51% cases vs. 20% controls, p < 0.001). The authors concluded that awkward postures are important predictors of symptoms that affect parts of the limb.

In a study comparing medical findings in full-time typists versus traditional office workers who rarely typed, Hunting et al. reported that abnormal medical findings, which were three times higher among the keyboard operators, were associated with awkward body postures.[37] For the data entry group, the incidence of pain due to isometric contraction of the right arm significantly increased (Mann Whitney U test, p < 0.01) when right ulnar deviation exceeded 20° and were less frequent when operators' hands and arms were supported.

In the cross-sectional survey of police transcribers, NIOSH performed a nested case-control follow-up evaluation of 10 subjects to identify potential risk factors for hand and wrist problems.[60] Five individuals with CTS or tendonitis were compared to five asymptomatic clerk/typists. Video analysis of typing demonstrated that the cases typed in greater wrist extensions (x = 24°, range = 15–30°) compared to controls (x = 16°, range = 0–25°). The authors suggested that the degree of wrist extension was controlled by the height of the chair relative to the keyboard surface, but they did not carry out statistical analysis to confirm their assumption.

Sauter et al. performed workstation evaluations of 40 VDT data entry workers.[59] Workstation characteristics and work postures that were hypothesized to influence upper and lower extremity and trunk discomfort were measured using a goniometer and a carpenter's level. Erect sitting postures and a higher backrest relative to the length of the operator's torso was associated with less frequent trunk discomfort. In the multiple regression model, higher keyboard height relative to elbow angle ($\beta = 0.31$, $R^2 = 0.1$) was a significant predictor for discomfort in both arms, and greater ulnar deviation of the right hand was associated with increasing discomfort on the right side.

A few years later, similar methods were used to examine a subset of 70 editors at a newspaper company.[24] Increasing neck rotation was associated with increasing neck and upper back symptoms. The authors also found that the effect of work postures on upper extremity symptoms was modified by psychosocial factors (see page 35).

In a questionnaire-based, cross-sectional study of 353 office workers by Bergqvist et al., nonneutral or extreme hand postures were found to be associated with arm/hand discomfort among computer users.[10] Moreover, individuals with ulnar deviation were shown to report discomfort.

In contrast to other studies, Starr et al. were unable to correlate static postural angles (e.g., neck, trunk, upper arm, forearm, hand, and elbow angles), measured by still photographs, with subjective reporting of physical discomfort among 100 VDT operators.[69] They suggested that the photographic technique may not be an adequate method to measure VDT posture variables, which are dynamic.

In all but one study, greater nonneutral postures (e.g., ulnar deviation, wrist extension, shoulder abduction, and flexion) have been identified as risk factors for musculoskeletal symptoms.[10,22,24,37,59,60]

Individual Risk Factors

A number of studies have reported an association between underlying systemic and physiologic disorders and an increased occurrence of MSD. Conditions such as rheumatic diseases and gout may lead to MSDs by triggering an inflammatory response of the synovium, leading to tenosynovitis and CTS. Conditions that lead to fluid imbalance, such as edema caused by pregnancy or obesity, can alter the pressure gradient between the neural vessels and surrounding tissues, causing nerve impairment.[71] These disorders and conditions may not lead to MSD symptoms themselves but, when combined with occupational exposures, may lead to MSDs.

GENDER

In their study of newspaper employees, Bernard et al. found that women were more likely than men to report neck (OR = 2.1, 95% CI = 1.4–2.4), shoulder (OR = 2.2, 95% CI = 1.5–3.3), and hand/wrist (OR = 1.7, 95% CI = 1.2–2.4) disorders.[8] When logistic regression analysis was restricted to jobs with comparable numbers of women and men, the odds ratios calculated for all regions remained similar to the original model, but gender differences were no longer statistically significant. Another NIOSH study of newspaper employees also found no significant gender difference when men and women performed comparable jobs.[16]

In a population-based study of occupational CTS using the Washington State Workers' Compensation database, Franklin et al. found no gender difference in 7,926 incident occupational CTS claims from 1984–1989.[25] The female-to-male ratio was 1.2:1 compared to 3:1 for nonoccupational CTS.[70]

In a prospective study of computer workers, Bergqvist et al. found that female gender was significantly associated with most upper extremity diagnoses in the univariate analyses.[11] In the final multivariate models, however, only "women with children at home" were found to be at significantly higher risk of hand/arm diagnoses (OR = 5.2, 95% CI = 1.2–22.8). The authors suggested that gender may therefore be a confounder for the nonoccupational risk factors more common in women. Child care and housekeeping were given as possible confounders, which were not usually examined or controlled for in most epidemiologic studies.

Based on these studies, female gender may not be an independent risk factor for MSDs but rather may confound for other nonwork-related factors or conditions commonly associated with women, such as the use of oral contraceptives, pregnancy, child care, and housekeeping. In addition, gender may act as a confounding factor for occupational exposures in which women are exposed to greater stresses than men. Small anthropometric dimensions (i.e., hand and height) may cause women to work in postures or at higher relative muscle forces, which cause greater mechanical stresses, than men.

ANTHROPOMETRY

Data on the influence of anthropometry on MSD symptoms are still lacking. Duncan and Ferguson found significant correlations ($p < 0.05$) between ulnar deviation and extension, shoulder flexion and wrist extension, and ulnar deviation among 90 teleprinters diagnosed with occupational cramps and myalgia.[22] In a study of 70 Australian keyboard operators, Green and Briggs examined height, weight, leg and arm lengths, biacromial width, upper and lower limb lengths, hip width, sitting and buttock-popliteal heights, and elbow-elbow breadth and found no anthropometric difference between eight men who reported MSD symptoms and 13 men who were symptom-free.[32] The small sample size for this group may have reduced the statistical power substantially. However, 27 women who reported MSD symptoms had wider hips (344.1 ± 29 mm) than 22 women who did not report symptoms (330.7 ± 16.6 mm) ($p = 0.05$). Comparison of body mass index (BMI = weight/height^2) between the two groups of women also suggested that, on average, symptomatic subjects (BMI = 26.2 ± 6.1) weighed more than the nonsymptomatic group (BMI = 23.2 ± 3.6).

Serina et al. conducted a laboratory study to evaluate the relationships between joint postures (i.e., wrist extension, ulnar deviation, and forearm pronation) and anthropometry (i.e., BMI, elbow height, hand length, shoulder width, wrist thickness, and width) in 25 healthy subjects who typed continuously for 10–15 minutes at a computer workstation.[61] In contrast to previous studies,[22,32] the authors found no significant correlation between wrist ulnar deviation and wrist extension, shoulder width, or BMI.

A few studies have addressed the potential role of anthropometry on MSDs. In an occupational setting, the lack of fit between anthropometry and equipment such as furniture or tools may lead to a worker's assuming nonneutral working postures, a risk factor for MSDs. Personal risk factors such as anthropometry cannot be controlled. Minimizing MSD risk factors will involve controlling potential determinants of postures, such as job designs and the geometry of the work objects, to accommodate workers whose personal factors predispose them to MSDs.

WORK ORGANIZATION AND PSYCHOSOCIAL FACTORS

Many studies have investigated the effects of work organization and psychosocial factors at work on the development of MSDs. Smith and Carayon suggest that work organization can contribute to MSD problems by defining the nature of work (i.e., repetition), establishing production standards (i.e., extent of exposures to MSD risk factors) and job/task designs (e.g., workstation, tools, and equipment used), setting work-rest cycles (e.g., work duration and work break frequency), defining the degree of work pressures, and providing a certain psychosocial climate for control over work decisions, job security, and socialization.[67] Thus, the definitions of work organization factors include aspects of the physical factors discussed above.

Cross-sectional studies of office workers have reported an association between psychosocial factors and MSD symptoms. Smith et al. used a questionnaire consisting of standardized job stress scales, psychological mood states, and frequency scales of health problems to investigate the influence of job stress on MSD complaints among 250 VDT workers.[67] Clerical VDT workers (data entry and retrieval clerks) reported significantly higher job stress and health problems than the professional VDT group (reporters, editors, and printers) or the controls who carried out the same tasks as the clerical VDT operators but did not use the VDT. Clerical VDT workers showed the highest level of stress and reported significantly more work pressure, less peer cohesion, and less autonomy than the other two groups. Significantly higher visual, musculoskeletal, and emotional health complaints were reported among the clerical VDT workers than the controls ($p < 0.05$). Thus, in this study, a relationship between job stress and health complaints exists.

Linton and Kamwendo reported significant associations between psychological work environment and neck and shoulder pains among 420 secretaries in a large medical center.[42] A series of questionnaires concerning the psychosocial work environment and musculoskeletal disorders were administered, and a psychosocial index was formed to define the best (good psychosocial environment) and worst (poor psychosocial environment) scores. Individuals who were exposed to "poor psychosocial environment" were about three times more likely to report neck (OR = 2.85, 95% CI = 1.28–6.32) and shoulder (OR = 3.32, 95% CI = 1.53–7.23) pain.

NIOSH cross-sectional studies of newspaper and telecommunication employees identified specific psychosocial factors to be associated with work-related MSD of the arm/wrist, forearm/elbow, shoulder, and neck regions.[34–35] Factors associated with the MSD symptoms included the following:

- hand and wrist—number of hours per week on deadline (OR = 4.4, 95% CI = 1.2–15.9) and less support from supervisors (OR = 1.5, 95% CI = 0.6–3.5)
- shoulders—less participation in the decision-making process (OR = 1.8, 95% CI = 0.7–4.9) and greater job pressure (OR = 1.7, 95% CI = 0.5–6.0)
- neck—number of hours per week on deadline (OR = 2.8, CI = 1.1–7.1), uneven workload during the workday (OR = 2.4, 95% CI = 0.9–6.9), and perception that management did not regard ergonomics as being important (OR = 2.3, 95% CI = 1.1–4.5).

In a NIOSH study of MSD prevalence at a telecommunications company, the following psychosocial variables were found to be significant predictors of upper extremity symptoms in logistic regression models:[35]

- hand and wrist—high information processing demands (OR = 2.3, 95% CI = 1.3–4.3

- shoulders—fear of being replaced by a computer (OR = 2.7, 95% CI = 1.4–5.8)
- elbow—fear of being replaced by computers (OR = 2.9, 95% CI = 1.4–6.1) perceived lack of decision-making opportunities (OR = 2.8, 95% CI = 1.4–5.7), and surges in workload (OR = 2.4, 95% CI = 1.2–5.0)
- neck—perceived lack of decision-making opportunities (OR = 4.2, 95% CI = 2.1–8.6), fear of being replaced by computers (OR = 3.0, 95% CI = 1.5–3.1), lack of productivity standard (OR = 3.5, 95% CI = 1.5–8.3), and increased work pressure (OR = 2.4, 95% CI = 1.1–5.5).

In the same study, symptom severity was found to be associated with increasing work pressure for all regions. Uncertainty about job future was associated with increased symptom severity in the neck, elbow, and hand/wrist. Lack of support from coworkers was associated with elbow symptoms, while lack of support from supervisors was associated with hand/wrist symptoms. The author suggested that social support may provide buffering to reduce negative effects of high work demands.

Faucett and Rempel reported interactions between psychosocial factors and work postures on reported musculoskeletal symptoms.[24] Using multiple regression analyses, they found that employees with poorer supervisory relationships reported greater symptom severity despite having better workstation ergonomics, defined as lower relative keyboard height and high seat back height ($R^2 = 0.1$, $p < 0.01$). As expected, workers with good supervisory relationships also reported less symptom severity and better workstation ergonomics ($R^2 = 0.05$, $p < 0.01$). The authors suggested that employees with poor supervisory relationships may be more likely to report increased symptoms, or their relationship may have deteriorated and persisted despite ergonomic improvement.

Current studies are based on self-reports of psychosocial variables and MSD symptoms. Objective measurements of physical loads are not often performed but are replaced with generic definitions, making it difficult to establish the relationship between physical and psychosocial factors. It is possible that as employees develop MSD symptoms, their productivity may be reduced, which in turn may cause them to experience increased stress and alterations in their relations with their coworkers and supervisors. Therefore, for cross-sectional studies, it is critical to estimate whether psychosocial or ergonomic variables are stable over time. Nonetheless, these studies provide some evidence that increasing work pressure and lack of job security or decision-making opportunities may contribute to the increased occurrence of work-related MSDs by modifying the type or extent of exposures to the risk factors or by modifying the individual responses to a given exposure.

In summary, computer-related risk factors demonstrating a consistent relationship with MSD include (1) computer use with sustained awkward postures, (2) long duration of computer use, and (3) work organization factors.

REFERENCES

1. Armstrong TJ, Chaffin DB: Some biomechanical aspects of the carpal tunnel. J Biomech 12:567–570, 1979.
2. Armstrong TJ: An Ergonomic Guide to Carpal Tunnel Syndrome. Akron, Ohio, American Industrial Hygiene Association, 1984.
3. Armstrong TJ, Fine LJ, Goldstein SA, et al: Ergonomics considerations in hand and wrist tendinitis. J Hand Surg 12A(part II):830–837, 1987.
4. Armstrong TJ, Buckle P, Fine LJ, et al: A conceptual model for work-related neck and upper limb musculoskeletal disorders. Scand J Work Environ Health 19:73–84, 1993.
5. Armstrong TJ, Foulke JA, Martin BJ, et al: Investigation of applied forces in alphanumeric keyboard work. Am Ind Hyg Assoc J 55:30–35, 1994.

6. Barnhart S, Demers PA, Miller M, et al: Carpal tunnel syndrome among ski manufacturing workers. Scand J Work Environ Health 17:46–52, 1991.
7. Bernard B, Sauter S, Peterson M, et al: Los Angeles Times. Cincinnati, National Institute for Occupational Health and Safety, 1993, HETA 90-013-2277.
8. Bernard B, Sauter S, Fine L, et al: Job task and psychosocial risk factors for work-related musculoskeletal disorders among newspaper employees. Scand J Work Environ Health 20:417–426, 1994.
9. Bergqvist U, Knave B, Voss M, Wibom R: A longitudinal study of VDT work and health. Int J Hum-Comp Int 4:197–219, 1992.
10. Bergqvist U, Wolgast E, Nilsson B, Voss M: Musculoskeletal disorders among visual display terminal workers: Individual, ergonomic and work organization factors. Ergonomics 38:763–776, 1995.
11. Bergqvist U, Wolgast E, Voss M: The influence of VDT work on musculoskeletal disorders. Ergonomics 38:754–762, 1995.
12. Borg G: Psychophysical scaling with applications in physical work and the perception of exertion. Scand J Work Environ Health 16:55–66, 1990.
13. Brown RA, Gelberman RH, Seiler JG, et al: Carpal tunnel release. A prospective, randomized assessment of open and endoscopic methods. J Bone Joint Surg 75A:1265–1275, 1993.
14. Buckle P: Work-related upper limb disorders amongst journalists. In Armstrong T (ed): Proceedings of the International Conference on Occupational Disorders of the Upper Extremities. Ann Arbor, MI, University of Michigan Center for Occupational Health and Safety Engineering, 1992.
15. Bureau of Labor Statistics: BLS Reports on Survey of Occupational Injuries and Illnesses in 1977–1995. Washington, DC, U.S. Department of Labor, 1995.
16. Burt S, Hornung R, Fine L, et al: Newsday Inc. Cincinnati, National Institute for Occupational Health and Safety, 1990, HETA 89-250-2046.
17. Cannon LJ, Bernacki EJ, Walter SD: Personal and occupational factors associated with carpal tunnel syndrome. J Occup Med 23:255–258, 1981.
18. Carragee EJ, Hentz VR: Repetitive trauma and nerve compression. Orthop Clin North Am 19:157–164, 1988.
19. Chiang HC, Ko YC, Chen SS, et al: Prevalence of shoulder and upper-limb disorders among workers in the fish-processing industry. Scand J Work Environ Health 19:126–131, 1993.
20. Chipman J, Kasdan M, Camacho D: Tendonitis of the upper extremity in occupational hand and upper extremity injuries and diseases. In Kasdan ML (ed): Occupational Hand & Upper Extremity Injuries and Diseases. Philadelphia, Hanley & Belfus, 1991, pp 412–418.
21. de Krom MCTFM, Kester ADM, Knipschild PD, Spaans F: Risk factors for carpal tunnel syndrome. Am J Epidemiol 132:1102–1110, 1990.
22. Duncan J, Ferguson D: Keyboard operating posture and symptoms in operating. Ergonomics 17:651–662, 1974.
23. Falck B, Aarnio P: Left-sided carpal tunnel syndrome in butchers. Scand J Work Environ Health 9:291–297, 1983.
24. Faucett J, Rempel DM: VDT-related musculoskeletal symptoms: Interactions between work posture and psychosocial work factors. Am J Ind Med 26:597–612, 1994.
25. Franklin GM, Haug J, Heyer N, et al: Occupational carpal tunnel syndrome in Washington State, 1984–1988. Am J Public Health 81:741–746, 1991.
26. Ferguson D: An Australian study of telegrahphist's cramp. Br J Ind Med 28:280–285, 1971.
27. Ferguson D, Duncan J: Keyboard design and operating posture. Ergonomics 17:731–744, 1974.
28. Gerard M, Armstrong T, Foulke J, et al: Effects of intra-subject typing speed on EMG, perceived exertion, and comfort while typing. Proceedings of the Prevention of Musculoskeletal Disorders Second Scientific Conference (PREMUS '95):143–145, 1995.
29. Gerr F, Letz T, Landrigan PJ: Upper-extremity musculoskeletal disorders of occupational origin. Annu Rev Public Health 12:543–566, 1991.
30. Goldstein SA, Armstrong TJ, Chaffin DB, Matthews LS: Analysis of cumulative strain in tendons and tendon sheaths. J Biomech 20:1–6, 1987.
31. Grandjean E, Nakaseko M, Hunting W, Laubli TH: Ergomische Untersuchugen zur entwichlung einer neuen tastatur fur buromaschinen (A new keyboard for office machines). Aeitschrift fur Arbeitowissenschaft 35:221–226, 1981.
32. Green RA, Briggs CA: Anthropometric dimensions and overuse injury among Australian keyboard operators. J Occup Med 31:747–750, 1991.
33. Hagberg M, Sudelin G: Discomfort and load on the upper trapezius muscle when operating a word processor. Ergonomics 29:1637–1645, 1986.
34. Hales TR, Sauter SL: US West Communications, Phoenix, AZ; Minneapolis, MN; Denver, CO. Cincinnati, National Institute for Occupational Health and Safety, 1992, HETA 89-299-2230.

35. Hales TR, Sauter SL, Peterson MR, et al: Musculoskeletal disorders among visual display terminal users in a telecommunications company. Ergonomics 37:1603–1621, 1994.
36. Hunting W, Laubli T, Grandjean E: Constrained postures in accounting machine operators. Appl Erg 11:145–149, 1980.
37. Hunting W, Laubli T, Grandjean E: Postural and visual loads at VDT workplace, Part 1: Constrained postures. Ergonomics 24:917–931, 1981.
38. Karasek R, Baker G, Marxer F, et al: Job decision latitude, job demands and cardiovascular disease: A prospective study of Swedish men. Am J Public Health 71:694–705, 1981.
39. Kendall D: Aetiology, diagnosis and treatment of paraesthesiae in the hands. Br Med J Clin Res 2:1633–1640, 1960.
40. Knave BG, Wilbom RI, Voss M, et al: Work with video display terminals among office employees. Scand J Work Environ Health 11:457–466, 1985.
41. Kuorinka I, Jonsson B, Kilbom A, et al: Standardized Nordic questionnaire for the analysis of musculoskeletal symptoms. Appl Erg 18:233–237, 1987.
42. Linton S, Kamwendo K: Psychosocial risk factors for neck and shoulder in secretaries. J Occup Med 31:609–613, 1989.
43. Luopajarvi T, Kuorinka I, Virolainen M, Holmberg M: Prevalence of tenosynovitis and other injuries of the upper extremities in repetitive work. Scand J Work Environ Health 5(suppl 3):48–55, 1979.
44. Maeda K, Hunting W, Grandjean E: Localized fatigue in accounting machine operators. J Occup Med 22:810–816, 1980.
45. Marcus M, Gerr F: Upper extremity musculoskeletal symptoms among female office workers: Associations with video display terminal use and occupational psychosocial stressors. Am J Ind Med 29:161–170, 1996.
46. Marras WS, Schoenmarklin RW: Wrist motions in industry. Ergonomics 36:341–351, 1993.
47. Moseley LH, Kalafut RM, Levinson PD, Mokris SA: Cumulative trauma disorders and compression neuropathies of the upper extremities. In Kasdan ML (ed): Occupational Hand and Upper Extremity Injuries and Diseases. 1st ed. Philadelphia, Hanley & Belfus, 1991.
48. Nathan PA, Meadow KD, Doyles LS: Occupation as a risk factor for impaired sensory conduction of the median nerve at the carpal tunnel. J Hand Surg 13:167–170, 1988.
49. Nathan PA, Keniston RC, Myers LD, Meadows KD: Obesity as a risk factor for slowing of sensory conduction of the median nerve in industry. A cross-sectional and longitudinal study involving 429 workers. J Occup Med 34:379–383, 1992.
50. National Institute for Occupational Safety and Health: Report of a Cross-Sectional Survey of Video Display Terminal Users at the Baltimore Sun, Baltimore, Maryland, Cincinnati, NIOSH, 1979, report PB83-195149.
51. National Institute for Occupational Safety and Health: Potential Health Hazard of Video Display Terminal: A NIOSH Research Report. Cincinnati, NIOSH, 1982, report 81-129.
52. Occupational Safety and Health Administration: Working Safely with Video Display Terminals. Washington, DC, U.S. Department of Labor, 1991, OSHA report 3092.
53. Phalen GS: The carpal-tunnel syndrome: Seventeen years' experience in diagnosis and treatment of six hundred fifty-four hands. J Bone Joint Surg 48A:211–228, 1966.
54. Punnett L: Work-related musculoskeletal disorders in computer keyboard operation. In Gordon S, Blair SJ, Fine L (eds): Repetitive Motion Disorders of the Upper Extremity. Rosemont, IL, American Academy of Orthopaedic Surgeons, 1995, pp 43–48.
55. Putz-Anderson P, Bernard B, Burt S, et al: Musculoskeletal Disorders and Workplace Factors: A Critical Review of Epidemiologic Evidence for Work-Related Musculoskeletal Disorders of the Neck, Upper Extremity, and Low Back. DHHS Pub No 97-141. Cincinnati, National Institute for Occupational Safety and Health, 1997.
56. Rempel DM, Harrison RJ, Barnhart S: Work-related cumulative trauma disorders of the upper extremity. JAMA 267:838–842, 1992.
57. Rempel D, Lopes J, Davila R, Davis B: Cumulative trauma among visual display terminal users at a newspaper company. Berkeley, CA, Health Hazard Evaluation System and Information Service, Department of Health Services, 1987.
58. Sabour M, Fadel H: The carpal tunnel syndrome, a new complication ascribed to the pill. Am J Obstet Gynecol 107:1265–1267, 1970.
59. Sauter SL, Schleifer LM, Knutson SJ: Work posture, workstation design, and musculoskeletal discomfort in a VDT data entry task. Hum Factors 33:151–167, 1991.
60. Seligman PJ, Boiano J, Anderson C: Minneapolis Police Department. Cincinnati, NIOSH, 1984, HETA 84-417-1745.
61. Serina ER, Tal R, Rempel D: Wrist and forearm postures and motions during typing. Ergonomics (in press).

62. Silverstein BA, Fine LJ, Armstrong TJ: Hand wrist cumulative trauma disorders in industry. Br J Ind Med 43:779–784, 1986.
63. Silverstein BA, Fine LJ, Armstrong TJ: Occupational factors and carpal tunnel syndrome. Am J Ind Med 11:343–358, 1987.
64. Silverstein BA: Prevalence of work-related musculoskeletal disorder symptoms in newspaper employees: Follow-up survey summary. In Armstrong T (ed): Proceedings of the International Conference on Occupational Disorders of the Upper Extremities. Ann Arbor, MI, University of Michigan Center for Occupational Health and Safety Engineering, 1992.
65. Smith EM, Sonstegard DA, Anderson WH: Carpal tunnel syndrome: Contribution of flexor tendons. Arch Phys Med Rehabil 58:379–385, 1977.
66. Smith MJ, Cohen BGF, Stammerjohn LW: An investigation of health complaints and job stress in video display operations. Hum Factors 23:387–400, 1981.
67. Smith MJ, Carayon P: Work organization, stress and cumulative trauma disorders. In Moon SD, Sauter SL (eds): Beyond Biomechanics: Psychosocial Aspects of Musculoskeletal Disorders in Office Work. London, Taylor and Francis, 1996, pp 23–41.
68. Starr SJ, Thompson CR, Shute SJ: Effects of video display terminals on telephone terminals on telephone operators. Hum Factors 24:699–711, 1982.
69. Starr SJ, Shute SJ, Thompson CR: Relating posture to discomfort in VDT use. J Occup Med 27:269–271, 1985.
70. Stevens JC, Sun S, Beard CM, et al: Carpal tunnel syndrome in Rochester, Minnesota, 1961–1980. Neurology 38:134–138, 1988.
71. Szabo SM, Madison M: Carpal tunnel syndrome as a work-related disorder. In Gordon S, Blair SJ, Fine L (eds): Repetitive Motion Disorders of the Upper Extremity. Rosemont, IL, American Academy of Orthopaedic Surgeons, 1995, pp 421–434.
72. Thompson DA: Effect of exercise breaks on musculoskeletal strain among data-entry operators: A case study. In Sauter S, Dainoff M, Smith M (eds): Promoting Health and Productivity in the Computerized Office-Models of Successful Ergonomic Interventions. New York, Taylor and Francis, 1990, pp 118–127.
73. Weislander G, Norback D, Gothe C, Juhlin L: Carpal tunnel syndrome (CTS) and exposure to vibration, repetitive wrist movements, and heavy manual work: A case-referent study. Br J Ind Med 46:43–47, 1989.

CHRISTINE B. NOVAK, PT, MS
SUSAN E. MACKINNON, MD

MULTIPLE NERVE ENTRAPMENT SYNDROMES IN OFFICE WORKERS

From the Division of Plastic and
  Reconstructive Surgery
Washington University School of
  Medicine
Program in Occupational Therapy
St. Louis, Missouri

Reprint requests to:
Christine B. Novak, PT, MS
Division of Plastic and
  Reconstructive Surgery
Suite 17424, East Pavilion
One Barnes-Jewish Hospital Plaza
St. Louis, MO 63144

In 1995, the Bureau of Labor Statistics reported more than 2 million lost-worktime injuries.[9a] This group included 31,457 cases of carpal tunnel syndrome, and 62% of the workers missed more than 21 days from work. Repetitive motion was associated with 99% of the carpal tunnel syndrome cases. Further analysis revealed that only 22% of the carpal tunnel syndrome cases were related to clerical work. In previously reported data from the Bureau of Labor Statistics, most carpal tunnel syndrome cases were associated with manufacturing jobs, such as meat packing, garment industries, motor vehicle manufacturing, and poultry processing.[31]

Reports of nerve compression syndromes have been increasing in frequency from both the private insurance industry and workers' compensation claims.[6,31,52] When these cases are labeled as work-related injuries, there is increased controversy surrounding the cause, diagnosis and treatment.[29,30,36,52,78,85] Nerve compression has been associated with exposure to physical stressors, including force, vibration, and position.[6,31] Increased duration of exposure to high force, vibration, and certain postures will increase the likelihood of developing carpal tunnel syndrome.[2,3,9,11,15,21,53,54,58,65,76,77] Jobs with high force, vibration exposure, and extreme wrist flexion/extension are more likely to be associated with carpal tunnel syndrome than jobs with low force, no vibration exposure, and minimal awkward positions. Because office work typically requires the latter, the causal association between office work and nerve compression has been extremely

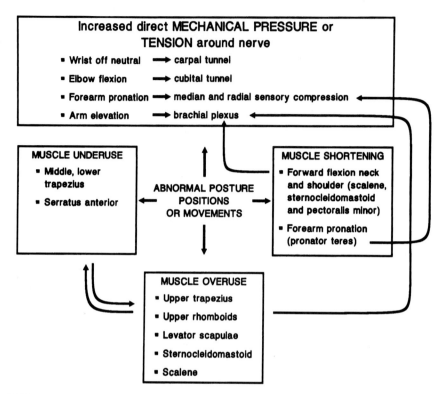

FIGURE 1. Hypothesis for multilevel nerve compression and muscle imbalance. (From Novak CB, Mackinnon SE: Thoracic outlet syndrome. Orthop Clin North Am 27:747–762, 1996; with permission.)

controversial. Nerve compression is unlikely to have a single cause, and its development depends not only on exposure to physical stressors but will be influenced by individual factors such as weight, age, and other associated medical conditions. Psychosocial issues also will influence the patient's perception of the management of the problem, particularly in work-related cases. We believe that multilevel nerve compression is a multifactorial problem whose successful management requires recognition of the multiple components.

HYPOTHESIS FOR MULTILEVEL NERVE COMPRESSION AND MUSCLE IMBALANCE

Prolonged postures or positions of the head, neck, and upper extremities that deviate from the ideal posture may contribute to complaints of pain, paresthesias, and numbness in the upper quadrant.[50] Maintaining these postures may have three major consequences (Fig. 1), as follows:

1. Certain postures or positions will place increased pressure on nerves by increasing pressure in entrapped nerve sites or by placing tension on nerves. Wrist flexion and extension have been shown to increase pressure within the carpal canal, thus increasing the pressure on the median nerve.[23,47,73,79,86] Similarly, elbow flexion will increase pressure within the cubital tunnel, which will cause increased pressure on the ulnar nerve.[67] The radial sensory nerve may be compressed between the tendons

of the brachioradialis and extensor carpi radialis longus with forearm pronation, and there will be increased stretch on the radial sensory nerve with added wrist flexion/ulnar deviation. Irritation of a nerve at an entrapment site may cause increased neural edema, inflammation, fibrosis, and decreased neural mobility. Neural blood supply may be further compromised by placing the nerve on tension—the median nerve with wrist extension, ulnar nerve with elbow flexion, and the brachial plexus with arm elevation.

2. These positions not only will place compression or tension on nerves but also will place muscles in shortened positions. Over time the muscles will undergo adaptive shortening.[27] When the muscle is stretched, the shortened muscle may produce local discomfort, and if the muscle crosses over a nerve, the nerve may be secondarily compressed (i.e., tightness of the pronator teres muscle causing compression of the median nerve in the forearm). Head-forward postures will place the scalenes, sternocleidomastoid, and suboccipital muscles in shortened positions. Initially, a more exaggerated head-forward position will decrease tension on these muscles. However, with prolonged positioning, the muscles will adaptively shorten and, then, with more upright postures, there will be increased tension and discomfort on the shortened muscles.

3. Abnormal postures and positions will cause some muscles to be positioned in elongated or shortened muscle lengths versus optimal musculoskeletal alignment. The muscles will undergo anatomic, biomechanical, and physiologic changes resulting in muscle weakness.[27] With weakness in some muscles, other muscles will be recruited to compensate for muscle underuse, and the cycle of muscle imbalance will continue. Head-forward and scapular abducted positions will result in elongation of the middle trapezius, lower trapezius, and shortening of the serratus anterior, scalenes, sternocleidomastoid, pectorals, and suboccipitals (Fig. 2). Weakness of the lower scapular stabilizers will result in the accessory use of the scapular elevators (upper trapezius, levator scapulae), thereby substituting scapular elevation for scapular rotation with glenohumeral flexion and abduction.

CHRONIC NERVE COMPRESSION

Symptoms resulting from chronic nerve compression are variable and range in the intensity and frequency of complaints. Understanding symptomatology requires an understanding of the histopathologic process in chronic nerve compression (Fig. 3). Compression of a sensory nerve will produce complaints that may vary from intermittent paresthesia to persistent numbness, while compression of a motor nerve may produce symptoms of aching, weakness, and muscle atrophy. These sensory and motor changes will parallel the spectrum of histopathologic changes that occur with chronic nerve compression.

Because surgical management of compression neuropathy is, at most, surgical decompression and it does not supply tissue for examination, there are few reports of the histopathology of nerve compression. Most studies investigating chronic nerve compression have used animal models, and the results have been extrapolated to humans.[46–49,64] Early patient complaints of intermittent paresthesia are likely a result of ischemia due to alteration in neural blood flow. The earliest histopathologic neural changes are seen in the blood-nerve-barrier (BNB) function. Following breakdown of the BNB function, there will be connective tissue thickening of both the internal and external epineurium. As the duration of compression increases, segmental demyelination will occur, causing focal nerve fiber changes and eventually diffuse demyelination. Finally, with diffuse changes and severe compression, axonal

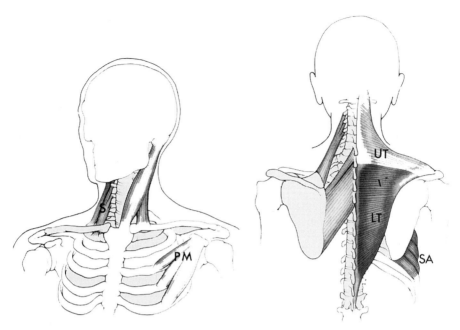

FIGURE 2.   Postural alterations from the ideal alignment frequently result in muscle imbalance in the cervicoscapular region. Tightness of the pectoralis minor (PM) and scalene (S) muscles may compress the brachial plexus. Weakness of the middle and lower trapezius (LT) and serratus anterior (SA) may cause overuse of the upper trapezius (UT) and levator scapulae. (From Mackinnon SE, Novak CB: Clinical commentary: Pathogenesis of cumulative trauma disorder. J Hand Surg 19A:873–883, 1994; with permission.)

degeneration will occur. The histopathologic changes that occur with chronic nerve compression will depend on the amount and duration of compression. With compression for a long period, the nerve will slowly progress through the spectrum of chronic nerve compression, but the changes may not occur uniformly across the nerve. Large fascicles in a nerve with a small amount of epineurium will be more susceptible to the effects of compression than will smaller fascicles surrounded by a large amount of epineurium.[38] Similarly, fascicles located more superficially will undergo changes due to the compression earlier than the fascicles located deeper within the nerve.[38] This may contribute to variable patient complaints within a single nerve distribution. Symptoms and clinical findings will progress with progression of the histopathologic changes. Experimentally, these changes occur slowly in animals; therefore, changes due to nerve compression in humans could progress over months or years.

Several entrapment sites in the upper extremity are commonly cited for their ability to compress the median nerve, ulnar nerve, radial nerve, and brachial plexus. The brachial plexus can be compressed between the anterior and middle scalene muscles as it passes over the first rib. The brachial plexus also can be compressed as it goes beneath the pectoralis minor muscle around the coracoid process. Distally, the median nerve can be compressed at the carpal tunnel or in the forearm by the pronator teres muscle. The ulnar nerve can be compressed at Guyon's canal, at the cubital tunnel, and at the lower trunk of the brachial plexus. The radial sensory nerve

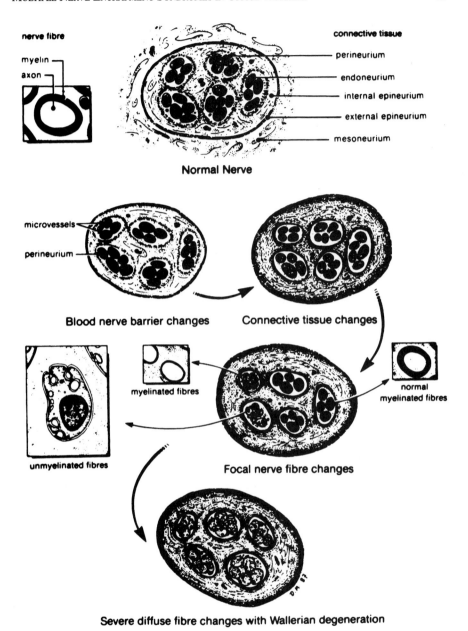

FIGURE 3. Histopathology of chronic nerve compression spans a range of changes from edema in the blood nerve barrier to axonal degeneration. The subjective complaints and clinical findings will parallel these histopathologic changes. (From Mackinnon SE, Dellon AL: Surgery of the Peripheral Nerve. New York, Thieme, 1988; with permission.)

can be compressed between the tendons of brachioradialis and the extensor carpi radialis longus. Compression of the radial nerve in the radial tunnel is less common and a more controversial diagnosis. Compression of the posterior interosseus nerve in the forearm will result in motor deficits only, although compression of motor afferents in the posterior interosseus nerve hypothetically may cause discomfort and pain. Knowledge of the sensory nerve distributions and motor nerve innervations will assist in identifying the involved nerve and the level of compression.[33,47]

In their double crush hypothesis, Upton and McComas proposed that a proximal level of nerve compression would render the more distal entrapment sites less tolerant to compressive forces.[83] Lundborg further expanded this concept by describing a reverse double crush, where distal nerve compression will affect more proximal nerve compressive sites.[38] Therefore, although each site in isolation may not be sufficient to produce symptoms or abnormalities with electrodiagnostic studies, multiple compression sites may together produce symptoms.[44] In patients with brachial plexus nerve compression, the summation of compressive forces may occur between the first rib and scalene muscles, beneath the clavicle, and beneath the pectoralis minor muscle around the coracoid process. This may then be combined with more distal nerve compression at the cubital tunnel or the carpal tunnel, causing complaints of paresthesia and numbness in the upper extremity with normal nerve conduction studies.

EVALUATION

Clinical evaluation will yield the most useful information regarding suspected chronic nerve compression, and therefore it is the most important aspect of the assessment.[44,47] Patient evaluation should begin with a detailed history, an assessment of subjective complaints, and a physical examination. The mechanism of injury, exacerbations, and previous treatment should be reviewed.

Subjective complaints resulting from chronic nerve compression will parallel the histopathologic changes (see Fig. 3). The subjective report of symptoms may vary between patients and even vary in different nerve distributions within a single patient depending on the severity of nerve compression. Initially, patients with compression of a sensory nerve will complain of intermittent paresthesia with prolonged positioning. This may in part explain the high prevalence of nocturnal symptoms, when patients are unaware of their positioning while sleeping. With more severe chronic nerve compression, more frequent paresthesia and numbness will be reported with less provocation, and, when axonal degeneration occurs, continuous numbness will be reported. Similarly, with compression of a motor nerve, patient complaints and clinical findings will vary. Initial complaints of aching will be followed by motor weakness and, finally, muscle atrophy. The muscle changes will occur with prolonged compression, and they are more likely to result from compression at more distal sites where the nerve is compressed between ligament and bony surfaces or tight fibrous bands. Proximal nerve compression of the brachial plexus is often accompanied by pain and discomfort. Therefore, patients will inherently alter their arm position to minimize discomfort and thus decrease the amount and duration of compression on the brachial plexus. This will decrease the progression of nerve compression to the more severe stages of nerve compression. Therefore, electrodiagnostic studies and sensibility tests remain normal.

Patients with more proximal nerve compression often complain of discomfort in the suprascapular, scapular, and cervical region with radiation of pain into the upper extremity. The pain is more likely of muscular origin than from nerve compression. Paresthesia and numbness may be isolated to a single nerve distribution (median, ulnar, or radial nerve), or sensory complains may include more than one nerve distribution. Compression of the brachial plexus may result in symptoms limited to the lower or upper trunk, but patients with long-standing symptoms, paresthesia, and numbness may describe symptoms that include the entire hand or upper extremity, particularly at night. Headaches in the occipital or orbital region may be reported.

The onset of symptoms is often described as insidious, or the patient may report a relatively minor trauma or a change in work pattern associated with a progressive increase in frequency and intensity of symptoms. For patients with diffuse upper extremity symptoms or long-standing complaints, further subjective evaluation using a pain questionnaire may be helpful. The pain evaluation questionnaire in use at our institution is a modification of the McGill pain questionnaire and Hendler's back screening questionnaire.[12,47] The modified questionnaire consists of a body diagram, a 10-cm visual analog scale for pain, stress, and coping; pain adjectives; and questions regarding home and work activities, onset, exacerbating factors, medications, and other factors. Each section is scored and labeled as positive if (1) more than three pain adjectives are selected, (2) the score on the questionnaire exceeds 20 points, or (3) the body diagram does not follow a known anatomic pattern. A positive score in two or three of the sections indicates that the pain is substantially impacting the patient's life. Such patients are referred for psychological or psychiatric assessment prior to any surgical intervention. The 10-cm visual analog scales do not affect the overall scoring, but they are more sensitive to change over time than the questionnaire and therefore can be used at subsequent visits to evaluate change with treatment.

Based on the concept of the double crush nerve compression, all potential sites of entrapment in the upper extremity should be assessed with tests of provocation (Table 1).[44,51] Clinical evaluation of the carpal tunnel using provocative maneuvers such as Phalen's test is well accepted, and this concept can be extrapolated to other entrapment sites.[20,42,61,66,68,69,91] In the earliest stages of chronic nerve compression, the provocative tests (position or pressure) will yield the most sensitive information to isolate each site of compression that is contributing to symptomatology. A Tinel's sign, using four to six digital taps on the nerve, is performed at each common nerve entrapment site in the upper extremity. It is considered positive with a sensory disturbance in the appropriate nerve distribution. Provocative maneuvers using positions of nerve tension or compression or direct pressure on the nerve are held for 1 minute. These maneuvers are considered positive with reproduction of symptoms in the appropriate neural distribution. When testing one entrapment site, care should be taken to avoid provocation at another site of potential nerve compression. The carpal tunnel is evaluated by placing the wrist in flexion and forearm in neutral (to avoid compression of the median nerve in the forearm by the pronator teres muscle). The examiner places digital compression on the median nerve just proximal to the distal wrist crease.[20,42,61,66,68,69,91] In this position of wrist flexion, the ulnar nerve at Guyon's canal may be compressed and, therefore, alteration of symptoms in the distribution of either the median or ulnar nerve should be recorded. The median nerve in the forearm is evaluated by placing the forearm in full supination with elbow extension and the wrist in a neutral position. Digital pressure is placed on the median nerve at the proximal border of the pronator teres muscle. The radial sensory nerve is provoked by placing the forearm in full pronation and the wrist in flexion with ulnar deviation. In this position, the extensor tendons in the first dorsal compartment are also stretched; therefore, DeQuervain's tenosynovitis should be considered in the differential diagnosis. The ulnar nerve at the cubital tunnel is provoked by placing the elbow in full flexion, wrist in neutral position, and digital pressure is placed on the

TABLE 1.   Provocative Tests for Nerve Entrapment

Nerve	Entrapment Site	Provocative Test	Management
Median nerve	Carpal tunnel	Pressure proximal to carpal tunnel Phalen's test Reverse Phalen's test (Hyperextension wrist)	Night splint wrist in neutral
	Proximal forearm	Pressure over proximal forearm in region of pronator teres Resisted elbow flexion, pronation and long finger flexion	Stretch pronator teres Rest periods in supination
Ulnar nerve	Guyon's canal	Pressure proximal to Guyon's canal	Night splint wrist in neutral
	Cubital tunnel	Elbow flexion and pressure proximal to cubital tunnel	Elbow pad Education: to decrease direct pressure on nerve and avoid elbow flexion
Radial nerve	Forearm	Pressure over junction of brachioradialis/extensor carpi radialis tendon Forearm pronation with wrist ulnar flexion	Positioning in supination and avoid repetitive pronation and supination activities
Brachial plexus	Supraclavicular and infraclavicular	Arm elevation above head Pressure over brachial plexus in interscalene region	Avoid arm elevated positions Postural correction Stretch shortened muscles and strengthen weakened scapular stabilizers

From Mackinnon SE, Novak CB: Evaluation of the patient with thoracic outlet syndrome. Semin Thorac Cardiovasc Surg 8:190–200, 1996; with permission.

ulnar nerve just proximal to the cubital tunnel.[60,67,70] In some patients, elbow flexion will cause the ulnar nerve to sublux anteriorly over the medial epicondyle; therefore, the examiner should evaluate the position of the ulnar nerve with elbow flexion to ensure that pressure is placed on the ulnar nerve.

The diagnosis for thoracic outlet syndrome (TOS) remains controversial, partially due to the subjective nature of the symptoms in patients with TOS.[13,14,88,89] The diagnosis should be based on subjective history, clinical examination, and exclusion of other causes of similar symptoms, such as cervical disc disease, nerve root impingement, shoulder pathology, cardiac conditions, esophageal conditions, pulmonary conditions, or space-occupying lesions such as tumors. By definition, TOS refers to compression of the neurovascular structures in the thoracic inlet.[75] In most patients with TOS, however, symptoms arise from compression of the brachial plexus as opposed to compression of the subclavian vein or artery.[75] The original tests for TOS, including Adson's test, Wright's maneuver, and shoulder retraction, were described to evaluate the integrity of the subclavian artery or vein, and they were considered to be positive with pulse obliteration of the radial artery. There have been reports of false positive and false negative findings with these tests.[75] This is particularly true in patients with neurogenic symptoms, in whom pulse obliteration, a measure of vascular insufficiency, would not be a good indicator of symptoms produced by brachial plexus nerve compression. Roos introduced a test of arm elevation with external rotation (AER) that requires patients to open and close their hands for 3 minutes in this arm-elevated position.[74] A positive response is noted with reproduction of symptoms. Sanders has reported positive findings with the 90° AER positioning and that the hand movements are not necessary.[75] Our test also uses the position of arm elevation, but we recommend elbow extension rather than elbow flexion to minimize irritation of the ulnar nerve at the cubital tunnel and wrist neutral position to minimize nerve provocation at the carpal canal.[51,62] The test is considered positive with reproduction of a patient's arm symptoms. Complaints of cervical or shoulder pain indicate the need for a more in-depth evaluation of the cervical spine or shoulder joint.

As nerve compression progresses, not only will tests of provocation be positive but sensory testing will become abnormal. Many tests and measurement tools have been described to evaluate sensibility, including tests evaluating tactile discrimination and threshold.[5,16–18,24,28,32,39–41,63,80] The different measurement tools likely evaluate different parameters of the sensory receptors located in the glabrous skin of the hand. The quickly adapting receptors (Pacinian and Meissner corpuscles) respond to movement, and the slowly adapting receptors (Merkel cell neurite complexes) respond to constant touch. Both tactile discrimination and threshold (minimum stimulus required to elicit a response) can be evaluated in the different types of receptors. Threshold of the slowly adapting receptors is assessed with cutaneous pressure thresholds and of the quickly adapting receptors with vibration thresholds.[4,5,17,28,32,39–41,63] Cutaneous pressure thresholds are often assessed using Semmes Weinstein monofilaments.[4,5] These nylon filaments vary in diameter and thus vary in the force applied to the skin. The subject indicates when a stimulus is applied, and the smallest filament that elicits a response is recorded as the cutaneous pressure threshold. Vibration thresholds are assessed subjectively with a 256-Hz tuning fork and quantitatively with a vibrometer.[17,28,32,39–41,63] Both single-frequency and multiple-frequency vibrometers are available to evaluate the minimal amplitude of vibration perceived.[17,19,28,32,39–41,63] Tactile discrimination is assessed with moving and static two-point discrimination (2pd).[17,18,63] The smallest spacing at which the patient can correctly distinguish two stimuli from one stimulus is recorded as the 2pd. Moving 2pd is assessed by moving the disk longitudinally from proximal to distal on the digit pulp, and static 2pd is evaluated by holding the disk stationary.[17,18,63] In the earlier stage of nerve compression, the measures of threshold will be most sensitive to changes that occur with nerve compression, and tests of tactile discrimination will remain normal. In the later stages with axonal degeneration, alterations in 2pd will be seen.

Strength measures are used to evaluate the motor system, and individual muscles can be tested to localize a problem to a specific nerve. Physical examination may be performed with manual muscle testing using the standard grades 0 to 5, or muscle strength can be quantified using commercially available manometers. However, because decreases in muscle strength due to nerve compression usually occur in the later stages of nerve compression, these measures will not be sensitive in the early stages.

Consequences of prolonged abnormal positions or postures are not restricted to the neural system but also affect the musculoskeletal system. Therefore, evaluation should include general observation of the patient sitting and standing and a more in-depth postural assessment.[33] In the ideal postural standing alignment, a plumb line dropped anterior to the lateral malleolus will fall anterior to the knee, through the greater trochanter, bisect the trunk, and fall midline to the shoulder, cervical spine, and ear. A head-forward, scapular abducted posture—the most common postural fault—involves head placement anterior to the thorax, thoracic flexion, scapular abduction, shoulder internal rotation, and alteration of cervical lordosis.

Postural misalignment will yield compensatory changes in muscle length and abnormal movement patterns. The muscles of the cervicoscapular region should be evaluated for abnormalities in movement patterns and individually for strength, length, spasm, and tenderness. Assessment of the shoulder should include the glenohumeral movements in addition to the associated scapular movements with shoulder flexion and abduction. Abnormalities of scapular position and movement can affect shoulder function, particularly the actions of rotator cuff muscles, and contribute to tendinitis or impingement.

Ancillary Tests

The diagnosis of nerve compression remains a clinical diagnosis, and ancillary tests should be used only to assist with the clinical diagnosis. Electrodiagnostic tests have been considered to be the gold standard for the diagnosis of nerve compression because they are objective. The use of motor and sensory latencies in median nerve compression at the level of the carpal tunnel has been well documented, as has ulnar nerve motor conduction velocities in patients with cubital tunnel syndrome. Urschel et al. have advocated using motor nerve conduction velocities to confirm the diagnosis of TOS, but these studies have been challenged.[47,75,84,88–90] Nerve conduction studies are useful in the diagnosis of distal nerve compression, but the value of these studies remains to be established in the diagnosis of brachial plexus nerve compression.

Other studies, including somatosensory evoked potentials (SSEP), radiographs, and computed tomography (CT), have been described in the diagnosis of TOS. Chest radiographs will reveal bony anomalies that may compress the neurovascular structures in the thoracic inlet, including cervical ribs and long transverse processes. Luoma et al. found CT helpful in identifying compression of the brachial plexus, but other studies have not found CT as useful.[7,62,75] Machleder et al. found SSEP abnormalities in 74% of 80 patients who were evaluated.[43] Yannikas and Walsh also found SSEP to be useful in the diagnosis of TOS.[92] Borg et al. suggested that stressed SSEP would be most useful in diagnosing TOS, because TOS tends to be a dynamic nerve compression syndrome.[8] We did not find dynamic SSEP helpful in the evaluation of our patients with TOS.[34] The diagnosis of neurogenic TOS remains a clinical diagnosis based on patient history, reproduction of symptoms with tests of provocation, and exclusion of other pathology. The value of magnetic resonance imaging in the diagnosis of TOS remains to be established.

MANAGEMENT

Management of patients with nerve compression must begin with patient education (Table 2). The patient requires an understanding of the problem, exacerbating and relieving positions, and strategies to minimize time spent in positions that exacerbate and perpetuate symptoms. For most patients, management requires modification of activities at home, work, and during sleep. We do not advocate cessation of work but, rather, alteration of work and nonwork activities.

Patients who awaken at night with pain, paresthesias, or numbness are provoking their symptoms by assuming awkward positions for prolonged times at night. Positions and patterns of sleep also should be addressed in patients who awaken in the morning with cervical stiffness or headaches. These patients will benefit from cervical support at night to protect the cervical spine from irritating positions. Prefabricated cervical collars are often recommended, but they will place most patients in excessive cervical extension. An alternative, cervical rolls, can be made

TABLE 2. Overview of Patient Management

A. Evaluation
  Nerve entrapment sites
  Posture
  Range of motion and movement patterns: cervical, scapula, shoulder, arm
  Exclude or identify other pathology: cervical disc disease, nerve root impingement, shoulder, tendinitis

B. Education
  Pathophysiologic process of single and multiple level nerve compression
    Positions of most risk and least risk for nerve compression
  Postural and positional correction
    Integration of corrected postures in activities of daily living at work, home, and sleep
  Impact of obesity, breast hypertrophy, and general physical condition

C. Treatment
  Postural and positional correction
    Neutral wrist splint at night, elbow pad, neck support for night use, lumbar support in sitting
  Physiotherapy
    Pain control and range of motion
      Stretching exercises for upper trapezius, levator scapulae, scalenes, sternocleidomastoid, pectorals, and chin retraction exercises (begin in supine with pillow support)
    Strengthening exercises for middle/lower trapezius, serratus anterior, lower rhomboids (begin in gravity assisted positions)
    Aerobic conditioning program
      Diaphragmatic and lateral costal breathing exercises
      Progressive walking program and other aerobic conditioning exercises
  Patient education and encouragement with compliance to home exercise program and behavior modification

From Novak CB, Collins ED, Mackinnon SE: Outcome following conservative management of thoracic outlet syndrome. J Hand Surg 20A:542–548, 1995; with permission.

from nonsterile composite padding and inserted into a 2-inch stockinette. Patients wear two rolls at night, and many report an immediate improvement in night and morning symptoms. However, some patients may require 1–2 weeks to become accustomed to these rolls. When night symptoms are under control, patients may then use commercially available pillow inserts for cervical support. Patients should be advised to avoid prone lying at night because of the excessive rotation and extension that is placed on the cervical spine.

Conservative management of carpal tunnel syndrome has been directed toward decreasing pressure in the carpal canal and thus decreasing pressure on the median nerve.[1,22,35,37,57,72] Patients are often told to wear wrist splints at night that position the wrist in extension. However, because wrist extension increases carpal canal pressure, this position will aggravate symptoms.[86] By contrast, splints that keep the wrist in a neutral position minimize carpal canal pressures. Therefore, these splints should be used at night, when most people assume a wrist flexed position. We do not advocate the use of splints during the day. A splint that maintains the wrist in a functional position of 30° extension will increase carpal canal pressures, and a splint in a neutral position to minimize carpal canal pressures will not be functional.[86] Splint use during repetitive hand motion has not been shown to reduce carpal canal pressures.[72] Patients should be informed about the risk of extreme wrist flexion/extension and strategies to minimize pressure on the median nerve at the wrist. Compression of the median nerve in the forearm is often relieved with stretching of the pronator teres muscle. Physical therapy modalities to treat chronic nerve compression, including carpal tunnel syndrome, have not been supported with efficacy studies.[1] Steroid injections have been reported in the conservative management of carpal tunnel syndrome but at best will give temporary relief and usually only in mild cases.[22]

Conservative management for radial sensory nerve compression requires patient education regarding positions that stretch or compress the radial sensory nerve (i.e., wrist flexion/ulnar deviation, tight watchbands and bracelets). Periodic stretching and positioning in forearm supination will decrease compression on the radial sensory nerve between the tendons of brachioradialis and the extensor carpi radialis longus. A steroid injection in this tendinous region may be useful, along with wearing a resting splint at night to maintain the wrist and thumb in a neutral position.

Cubital tunnel syndrome is hypothesized to result from compression and tension on the ulnar nerve at the medial epicondyle with elbow flexion or as the ulnar nerve enters between the two heads of the flexor carpi ulnaris muscle. Conservative management should begin with patient education regarding elbow flexion and compression of the ulnar nerve in this position. Patients should be instructed to minimize flexed elbow postures. We recommend using elbow pads at night and teaching patients to go into elbow extension when they awaken at night. Elbow extension splints are rarely tolerated by patients at night and therefore show poor patient compliance. Stretching of the flexor carpi ulnaris muscle will be useful in cases where most of the compression on the ulnar nerve is distally at this muscle.

Therapy will play the greatest role with conservative management of TOS. Night symptoms can be controlled in most patients with cervical rolls. Complaints of pain, paresthesia, and numbness likely result from nerve compression and musculoskeletal imbalances. Therefore, treating only the nerve compression will not totally relieve symptoms. Postural faults in the cervicoscapular region will cause alteration of cervical and scapular mobility. This altered mobility will have consequences not only in the cervicoscapular region but also may refer symptoms distally into the upper extremity. Trunk positions will affect the cervical, thoracic, and lumbar spine and the extremities. Therefore, a complete postural evaluation is necessary.[33] Postural alignment should be assessed in standing and sitting positions and should be compared to the ideal posture. Initially, many patients will not tolerate postural correction into the ideal position because excessive tension will exist on tight structures (Fig. 4). Such patients require stretching exercises to comfortably achieve these positions and then strengthening exercises to maintain them.

Mobility of the cervical spine can be achieved using the approach outlined by McKenzie.[55] He cites three factors that are relevant to patients with TOS: bad sitting posture, increased frequency of flexion, and loss of cervical lordosis, which will lead to tight cervical structures and thus to cervical restriction. Cervical retraction exercises are used to stretch the tight restrictive structures and to increase cervical mobility. Initially, repetition of cervical retraction should produce a decrease of discomfort or symptom centralization. If this is not reported by the patient, the retraction exercises should begin in a supine position with the head and neck supported on a pillow. With decreased discomfort, the degree of cervical flexion is decreased by removing the pillow, and the patient is then taught exercises to achieve full cervical retraction in lying and sitting. With full cervical retraction, the exercises then progress to full cervical extension, as outlined by McKenzie.[55,56]

Evaluation of the cervical spine, shoulder, and scapula is necessary to identify abnormal movement patterns and the muscles contributing to these patterns. Faulty postural alignment will result in some muscles being placed in elongated positions, thus placing them at a mechanical disadvantage, and other muscles will act in

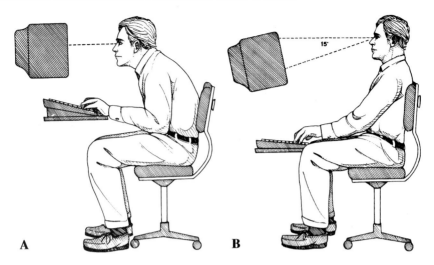

FIGURE 4. *A*, Improper posture at the computer results in head/neck/shoulder forward positions. *B*, A keyboard that is placed lower will decrease scapular elevation and elbow flexion. Adequate chair support is necessary to maintain an upright posture. The addition of a wrist support can cause direct pressure on the median nerve and therefore should be used with caution. (From Mackinnon SE, Novak CB: Clinical commentary: Pathogenesis of cumulative trauma disorder. J Hand Surg 19A:873–883, 1994; with permission.)

shortened positions.[87] Typical positions (head forward, thoracic flexed, scapulae abducted, and shoulders internally rotated) will result in elongation of the middle trapezius and lower trapezius and tightness of the upper trapezius, serratus anterior, scalenes, sternocleidomastoid, and suboccipitals. With elongation and weakness of the middle and lower trapezius there will be overuse of the muscles that assist with scapular elevation, including the upper trapezius, levator scapulae, and upper rhomboids. The cycle of muscle imbalance substituting scapular elevation for scapular rotation with glenohumeral movements will continue until muscle balance is achieved. Therefore, successful conservative management depends on the restoration of muscle balance in the cervicoscapular region. Muscles that are decreased in length should be palpated for tenderness and trigger points. These hyperirritable regions can cause local discomfort or refer pain distally in patterns as described by Travell and Simons.[82] Mechanical irritants, such as abnormal postures, can stimulate the trigger points and thus perpetuate local discomfort or distally referred pain. It is therefore necessary to restore muscle length. A number of techniques have been described to help achieve full muscle length. Effective stretching must begin at patient tolerance, because aggressive stretching will needlessly exacerbate symptoms and likely cause increased muscle spasm. Stretches that are held longer (at least 15 seconds) will be most effective in regaining muscle length and decreasing trigger point activity. If stretching in isolation does not decrease discomfort and increase muscle length, the stretching can be augmented with a vapocoolant spray as described by Travell and Simons.[82] As muscle irritability decreases, more aggressive stretching can be implemented. In most cases, specific stretching will begin with stretches for the upper trapezius, levator scapulae, and pectorals. The cervical retractions will stretch the suboccipitals, sternocleidomastoid, and scalene muscles. Stretching the pectoralis major using a "corner stretch" should be avoided initially, because most

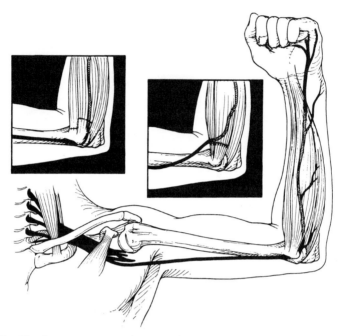

FIGURE 5. The "corner stretch" will place the brachial plexus on maximal stretch, and with added elbow flexion, tension will be placed on the ulnar nerve. Stretches in this region should be given with consideration of the neural structures. An anterior transposition as shown in the boxes will relieve tension on the ulnar nerve and, hypothetically, on the entire neural line. (From Mackinnon SE, Novak CB: Clinical commentary: Pathogenesis of cumulative trauma disorder. J Hand Surg 19A:873–883, 1994; with permission.)

patients will not tolerate a full stretch to this region. In this position, the neural structures are placed on stretch through the brachial plexus and, with the addition of elbow flexion, there is added stretch to the ulnar nerve (Fig. 5). Excessive tension on the entire neural line will likely exacerbate symptoms throughout the entire upper extremity. However, neural mobility and length are necessary for full upper extremity painfree range of motion. Knowledge of neural tension testing and problems associated with overstretching neural tissues is important in the treatment of patients with proximal upper extremity nerve compression.[10,81] Most of these patients must begin with segmental stretches over one joint and progress to more complex stretches over multiple joints, as tolerated.[81]

Conservative management of patients with proximal-level nerve compression and cervicoscapular muscle imbalance must be directed toward the restoration of muscle balance. In most patients, the correction of muscle imbalance can be achieved with an exercise program without physical therapy modalities.[59] Physical therapy modalities should be used sparingly in these patients, especially if they encourage dependence on therapy. Thermal agents, iontophoresis, ultrasound, and transcutaneous electrical nerve stimulation may be used for temporary pain relief if necessary for patient compliance to the exercises. These modalities should not be considered as an alternative to an appropriate exercise program. They only give temporary pain relief, and long-term pain relief can be obtained only by correcting abnormal movement patterns and muscle balance.

With improvement in cervical movement, scapular mobility, and relative pain control, a muscle strengthening exercise program can begin. General resisted strengthening exercises will not correct muscle imbalance because the stronger muscles will continue to be incorrectly recruited. The exercises also are likely to exacerbate pain in the cervicoscapular region. Individual muscle assessment is necessary to determine which muscles are weak. Strengthening exercises should begin in gravity-assisted positions in most patients, but some patients may require gravity-eliminated positions. Strengthening is usually targeted to the weak middle trapezius, lower trapezius, and serratus anterior muscles to decrease compensatory overuse of the scapular elevators (upper trapezius and levator scapulae). Strengthening of the lower scapular stabilizers in a gravity-eliminated position will begin in side-lying to permit correct recruitment of these muscles without compensation of the scapular elevators. As scapular rotation improves with glenohumeral flexion, the patient is progressed to gravity-assisted positions, then to exercises against gravity, and finally to exercises with resistance. Emphasis should be placed on correct muscle recruitment and muscle endurance rather than muscle power.

Obesity and poor physical condition have been associated with nerve compression. Poor aerobic conditioning will cause secondary respiratory muscles to be used even during quiet respiration. The accessory respiratory muscles, including the scalenes, sternocleidomastoid, and upper trapezius, will become hypertrophied with excessive use and may undergo adaptive shortening if postured in a shortened position.[71] Tightness and hypertrophy of the scalene muscles will compress the brachial plexus between the anterior scalene, the middle scalene, and the first rib. To decrease excessive use of the accessory respiratory muscles and to increase the efficiency of the respiratory system, patients should assume a more upright posture to decrease thoracic flexion and thus increase chest expansion with inspiration. Patients also should be taught diaphragmatic and lateral costal breathing exercises. An aerobic exercise program is necessary to improve the cardiovascular system. Most programs begin with walking using a correct breathing pattern. When introducing other types of aerobic exercise, attention should be paid to the head and arm position to avoid excessive cervical extension or head-forward positions and to avoid excessive loading of the arms.

Suggestions and referrals are frequently made for orthotic supports to achieve upright postures. These supports often have straps that are positioned anterior to the shoulder and then cross to the back in a figure-eight pattern. The straps can place excessive pressure over the brachial plexus and the pectoralis minor and cause increased discomfort. The desired upright postures can and should be achieved with an appropriate stretching exercise program and then maintained with increased strength of the lower scapular stabilizers and thoracic extensor muscles. Women with breast hypertrophy may benefit from a bra that crosses in the back to remove the load of the bra strap from the suprascapular region and to encourage a more upright posture. In some cases, a reduction mammoplasty is successful in reducing symptoms.[26]

The problem of obesity must be addressed from the direct effect on nerve compression and from the excessive load on the brachial plexus. In a recent outcome study of patients with multilevel nerve compression, obesity was a significant factor in unsuccessful conservative management.[59] Obese patients should be directed to a nutritionist or weight loss program to obtain a suitable diet and exercise program.

SURGICAL MANAGEMENT

Surgical intervention for multilevel nerve compression should be offered only to patients in whom conservative treatment was unsuccessful. To avoid disappointment, the patient and surgeon must have realistic expectations regarding the symptoms that may be alleviated with surgery. Clearly, a carpal tunnel release will not relieve most symptoms in patients with multilevel nerve compression and cervicoscapular muscle imbalance. A carpal tunnel release will decompress the median nerve and relieve symptoms only in the median nerve distribution of the hand. Therefore, patients expecting total relief of symptoms in the upper extremity will view the carpal tunnel release as a failure even if paresthesia and numbness are no longer present in the median nerve distribution.

Carpal tunnel release to decompress the median nerve has been described using a number of surgical techniques, including an open technique, endoscopy with single and double portals, and a limited incision approach. We prefer an open technique and have found no problems with scar tenderness or return-to-work issues that are occasionally ascribed to this technique. The surgery is performed under an intravenous regional block using an arm tourniquet. To prevent postoperative sympathetic pain, 1.5 ml/kg of bretylium is added to the intravenous solution when pain is a significant component of the patient's symptomatology. A standard longitudinal incision is made well ulnar to the thenar crease. If necessary, the incision can be extended proximally past the distal wrist crease in a zigzag fashion for complete decompression of the median nerve by release of the antebrachial fascia. Blunt dissection, protecting the cutaneous sensory nerves, is carried out to expose the transverse carpal ligament. The ligament is then divided in a proximal-to-distal direction, and the antebrachial fascia is released under direct vision. A long-acting anesthetic agent such as Marcaine is used for postoperative patient comfort, and a bulky dressing is applied to maintain the wrist in a neutral position. About 2–3 days postoperatively, the bulky dressing is removed, and the patient is taught range of motion exercises for the hand, wrist, elbow, and shoulder. A wrist resting splint is used at night for about 3 weeks to provide comfort.

A number of surgical techniques have been described for the treatment of ulnar nerve compression at the cubital tunnel, including simple decompression, medial epicondylectomy, and anterior transposition of the ulnar nerve, placing it subcutaneously, submuscularly, or intramuscularly. We recommend an anterior submuscular transposition for complete decompression of the ulnar nerve in both elbow flexion and extension.[45] A step-lengthening of the antebrachial fascia is performed. Frequently, the patient has a large enough flexor/pronator muscle mass that the proximal dissection is at the level of the brachialis muscle but the distal dissection is only at an intramuscular level. Bipolar cautery, 4.5 loupe magnification, and a portable nerve stimulator are used during the procedure. With the patient in an arm tourniquet and under an axillary block or continuous intravenous regional anesthetic,[25] an incision is made posterior to the medial epicondyle, over the ulnar nerve. Care is taken to protect any branches of the medial antebrachial cutaneous nerve (MABC) that may cross the incision. If a branch of the MABC nerve is inadvertently cut, it is turned back into the proximal muscle bed to prevent a painful neuroma or scar. The ulnar nerve is identified posterior to the medial intermuscular septum, and it is encircled with umbilical tape, taking care to avoid traction on the nerve. The ulnar nerve is then released proximally, including the brachial fascia. The medial intermuscular septum is excised about 5–7 cm proximal to the medial epicondyle. The nerve is then followed distally through the cubital tunnel, releasing fascial or muscular attachments from the medial epicondyle. A thickened Osborn's band is often identified at the proximal edge of the flexor carpi ulnaris muscle, and it is released, as is the fascial tissue between the two heads of the flexor carpi ulnaris. The fascial tissue should be released as far distally as necessary to ensure a smooth anterior transposition of the ulnar nerve. A subcutaneous flap is raised on the fascia of the flexor/pronator origin, and the ulnar nerve is gently transposed anteriorly to evaluate its position. The small posterior motor nerve branches to the flexor carpi ulnaris and/or flexor digitorum profundus, which may tether the nerve posteriorly, are carefully dissected away from the main ulnar nerve. The flexor/pronator fascia is cut in a step-lengthened fashion, and the fascial flaps are elevated from the muscle. The dissection is continued down to the brachialis muscle proximally, and distally the dissection is deep enough to allow good coverage of the ulnar nerve. Tendinous bands in the flexor/pronator muscle mass are excised so that they do not compress the ulnar nerve. The ulnar nerve when transposed anteriorly will lie on the brachialis muscle adjacent to the median nerve. Any additional fascia should be released to ensure that the ulnar nerve is completely decompressed, proximally and distally. A suction drain is placed at the incision site and removed the next day. The fascia of the flexor origin is closed in a lengthened position with 4-0 nonabsorbable sutures. A long-acting anesthetic is placed at the incision to minimize postoperative discomfort. The incision is then closed with subcuticular absorbable sutures and steri-strips. A bulky dressing using a fiberglass backslab is applied to maintain elbow flexion, the forearm in neutral, and the wrist in neutral. This dressing is removed 2–3 days postoperatively, and the patient is given a sling to wear at night and occasionally during the day as desired. The patient is instructed in range of motion for the hand, wrist, elbow, and shoulder and cautioned to gently move the arm into full elbow supination and extension. This early mobilization of the extremity is extremely important to minimize adhesions and to promote optimal neural mobility. Full active range of motion, including elbow extension with full forearm supination, is expected within 3–4 weeks. Light resistive/strengthening exercises and loading of the extremity may begin after 4 weeks and progress as tolerated by the patient.

Surgical management of neurogenic TOS with no muscle atrophy should be offered only to patients in whom conservative management has failed and who have attempted to modify work, home, and personal factors such as weight loss but continue to be significantly affected by the symptoms. A surgical approach through a supraclavicular incision provides good visualization for protection of all structures during decompression of the brachial plexus, release of the scalenes, and excision of the first rib. Microbipolar cautery, 4.5 loupe magnification, and a portable nerve stimulator are used during surgery. With a sandbag between the scapulae and the neck extended to the nonoperative side, an incision is made 2 cm above and parallel to the clavicle in the supraclavicular fossa. The supraclavicular nerves are identified beneath the platysma and mobilized to permit vessel loop retraction. The omohyoid muscle is divided and the supraclavicular fat pad elevated. The lateral portion of the clavicular head of the sternocleidomastoid is divided and will be repaired at the end of the surgical procedure. The phrenic nerve is seen on the anterior surface of the anterior scalene muscle, and the long thoracic nerve is seen on the posterior aspect of the middle scalene muscle. Both of these nerves should be visualized and protected throughout the procedure. The anterior scalene muscle is divided from the first rib. The subclavian artery is seen behind the anterior scalene muscle and is encircled with umbilical tape. The brachial plexus nerve trunks are visualized and gently mobilized. The middle scalene muscle is divided from the first rib, and care should be taken to avoid injury to the long thoracic nerve that may have branches through or posterior to the middle scalene muscle. The brachial plexus is visualized, and the lower trunk and the C8–T1 nerve root are identified above and below the first rib. Congenital bands and Sibson's fascia are divided. The first rib is encircled and, where it is easily visible, is divided with bone-cutting instruments. Using a rongeur, the posterior segment of the rib is removed extending back to the cartilaginous components of the articular facets, and the anterior segment of the rib is removed to the costosternal cartilaginous attachment. Cervical ribs or long transverse processes are removed using a similar technique. The pleura is opened at the superior dome to allow drainage of any postoperative blood into the chest cavity rather than allowing it to collect around the brachial plexus. Care should be taken to protect the intercostal brachial nerve when opening the pleura. A long-acting local anesthetic is placed in the incision and around the brachial plexus to assist with postoperative comfort. The wound is closed in a subcuticular fashion, and a simple suction drain is used and sealed after wound closure and after maximal lung inflation. On the day after surgery, the patient is taught gentle range of motion exercises of the cervical spine and upper extremity. The patient is given soft cervical rolls for night use. Desensitization and massage at the incision will help to decrease hypersensitivity and is encouraged beginning in the first postoperative week. Full range of motion is expected by 4 weeks following surgery, and supervised therapy may then be recommended to increase strength and maintain painless range of motion. Releasing the scalene muscles and excising the first rib will decompress the brachial plexus but will not affect the problems associated with muscle imbalance. Therefore, specific strengthening of muscles in the cervicoscapular may be necessary following surgery. Work conditioning or work hardening is usually necessary only for patients who are heavy laborers or who have not worked for a long time prior to surgery.

Multilevel nerve compression in office workers is treatable and compatible with work and should not cause permanent disability. A great deal of emphasis in the management of work-related musculoskeletal complaints has been directed toward alteration of the work environment. We believe that successful management of the office worker with nerve compression begins with the patient's understanding of the problem. This is a multifactorial problem involving personal, physical, and psychological factors. Changing only the work component of this paradigm will not yield a successful outcome, particularly in patients with multilevel nerve compression and cervicoscapular muscle imbalance. The many factors associated with this problem must be identified for optimal management. The individual must comply with an appropriate exercise program and also make the necessary changes at home, in the workplace, and in personal factors for a successful outcome.

REFERENCES

1. Banta CA: A prospective nonrandomized study of iontophoresis, wrist splinting and antiinflammatory medication in the treatment of early-mild carpal tunnel. J Occup Med 36:166–168, 1994.
2. Barnhart S, Demers PA, Miller M, et al: Carpal tunnel syndrome among ski manufacturing workers. Scand J Work Environ Health 17:46–52, 1991.
3. Baron S, Milliron M, Habes D, et al: Shoprite Supermarkets. Cincinnati, National Institute for Occupational Safety and Health, 1991, NIOSH HETA report 88-344-2092.
4. Bell-Krotoski JA: Sensibility testing: Current concepts. In Hunter JM, Mackin EJ, Callahan AD (eds): Rehabilitation of the Hand: Surgery & Therapy. St. Louis, Mosby, 1995, pp 109–128.
5. Bell-Krotoski JA, Weinstein S, Weinstein C: Testing sensibility, including touch-pressure, two-point discrimination, point localization and vibration. J Hand Ther 6:114–123, 1993.
6. Bernard BP: Musculoskeletal disorders and workplace factors. Cincinnati, U.S. Department of Health and Human Services, 1997, DHHS (NIOSH) publication 97-141.
7. Bilbey JH, Muller NL, Connell DG, et al: Thoracic outlet syndrome: Evaluation with CT. Radiology 171:381–384, 1989.

8. Borg K, Persson HE, Lindblom U: Thoracic outlet syndrome: Diagnostic value of sensibility testing, vibratory thresholds and somatosensory evoked potentials at rest and during perturbation with abduction and external rotation of the arm. Proceedings of the World Congress on Pain, Amsterdam I:144–150, 1988.

9. Bovenzi M: Italian study group on physical hazards in the stone industry: Hand-arm vibration syndrome and dose-response relation for vibration-induced white finger among quarry drillers and stonecarvers. Occup Environ Med 51:603–611, 1994.

9a. Bureau of Labor Statistics, USDL 97-188, Washington, DC, United States Department of Labor, 1997.

10. Butler DS: Mobilisation of the Nervous System. Melbourne, Churchill Livingstone, 1991.

11. Cannon LJ, Bernacki EJ, Walter SD: Personal and occupational factors associated with CTS. J Occup Med 23:255–258, 1981.

12. Chen DL, Novak CB, Mackinnon SE, Weisenborn SA: Pain responses in patients with upper-extremity disorders. J Hand Surg 2:70–75, 1998.

13. Cherington M, Cherington C: Thoracic outlet syndrome: Reimbursement patterns and patient profiles. Neurology 42:943–945, 1992.

14. Chernington M, Happer I: Surgery for thoracic outlet syndrome may be hazardous to your health. Muscle Nerve 9:632–634, 1986.

15. Chiang H, Chen S, Yu H, Ko Y: The occurrence of carpal tunnel syndrome in frozen food factory employees. Kao Hsiung I Hsueh Ko Hsueh Tsa Chih 6:73–80, 1990.

16. Dellon AL: Clinical use of vibratory stimuli to evaluate peripheral nerve injury and compression neuropathy. Plast Reconstr Surg 65:466–476, 1980.

17. Dellon AL: Evaluation of Sensibility and Re-education of Sensation in the Hand. Baltimore, Williams & Wilkins, 1981.

18. Dellon AL, Mackinnon SE, Crosby PM: Reliability of two-point discrimination measurements. J Hand Surg 12A:693–696, 1987.

19. Doezie AM, Freehill AK, Novak CB, Mackinnon SE: Evaluation of vibration thresholds in medical transcriptionists. J Hand Surg 22A:867–872, 1997.

20. Durkan J: A new diagnostic test for carpal tunnel syndrome. J Bone Joint Surg 73A:535–538, 1997.

21. Feldman RG, Travers PH, Chirico-Post J, Keyserling WM: Risk assessment in electronic assembly workers: Carpal tunnel syndrome. J Hand Surg 12A:849–855, 1987.

22. Gelberman RH, Aronson D, Weisman MH: Carpal tunnel syndrome: Results of a prospective trial of steroid injection and splinting. J Bone Joint Surg 62A:1181–1184, 1980.

23. Gelberman RH, Hergenroeder PT, Hargens AR, et al: The carpal tunnel syndrome: A study of carpal tunnel pressures. J Bone Joint Surg 63A:380–383, 1981.

24. Gelberman RH, Szabo RM, Williamson RV, Dimick MP: Sensibility testing in peripheral-nerve compression syndromes. J Bone Joint Surg 65A:632–638, 1983.

25. Glickman LT, Mackinnon SE, Rao TV, McCabe SJ: Continuous intravenous regional anesthesia. J Hand Surg 17:82–86, 1992.

26. Gonzalez F, Walton RL, Shafer B, et al: Reduction mammaplasty improves symptoms of macromastia. Plast Reconstr Surg 91:1270–1276, 1993.

27. Grossman MR, Sahrmann SA, Rose SJ: Review of length-associated changes in muscle. Phys Ther 62:1799–1808, 1982.

28. Grunert BK, Wertsch JJ, Matloub HS, McCallum-Burke S: Reliability of sensory threshold measurement using a digital vibrogram. J Occup Med 32:100–102, 1990.

29. Hadler NM: A keyboard for "Daubert" [editorial]. J Occup Environ Med 38:469–476, 1996.

30. Hadler NM: Repetitive upper extremity motions in the workplace are not hazardous. J Hand Surg 22A:19–29, 1997.

31. Hales TR, Bernard BP: Epidemiology of work-related musculoskeletal disorders. Orthop Clin North Am 27:679–710, 1996.

32. Jetzer T: Use of vibration testing in the early evaluation of workers with carpal tunnel syndrome. J Occup Med 33:117–120, 1991.

33. Kendall FP, McCreary EK, Provance PG: Muscles: Testing and Function. Baltimore, Williams & Wilkins, 1993.

34. Komanetsky RM, Novak CB, Mackinnon SE, et al: Somatosensory evoked potentials fail to diagnose thoracic outlet syndrome. J Hand Surg 21A:662–666, 1996.

35. Kruger VL, Kraft GH, Deitz JC, et al: Carpal tunnel syndrome: Objective measures and splint use. Arch Phys Med Rehabil 72:517–520, 1991.

36. Lister GD: Ergonomic disorders. J Hand Surg 20A:353, 1995.

37. Luchetti R, Schoenhuber R, Alfarano M, et al: Serial overnight recordings of intracarpal canal pressure in carpal tunnel syndrome patients with and without wrist splinting. J Hand Surg 19B:35–37, 1994.

38. Lundborg G: Nerve Injury and Repair. New York, Churchill Livingstone, 1988.
39. Lundborg G, Dahlin LB, Lundstrom R, et al: Vibrotactile function of the hand in compression and vibration-induced neuropathy. Scand J Plast Reconstr Hand Surg 25:1–5, 1992.
40. Lundborg G, Lie-Stenstrom A, Stromberg T, Pyykko I: Digital vibrogram: A new diagnostic tool for sensory testing in compression neuropathy. J Hand Surg 11A:693–699, 1986.
41. Lundborg G, Sollerman C, Stromberg T, et al: A new principle for assessing vibrotactile sense in vibration-induced neuropathy. Scand J Work Environ Health 13:375–379, 1987.
42. MacDermid J: Accuracy of clinical tests used in the detection of carpal tunnel syndrome: A literature review. J Hand Ther 4:169–176, 1991.
43. Machleder HI, Moll F, Nuwer M, Jordan S: Somatosensory evoked potentials in the assessment of thoracic outlet syndrome. J Vasc Surg 6:177–184, 1987.
44. Mackinnon SE: Double and multiple crush syndromes. Hand Clin 8:369–380, 1992.
45. Mackinnon SE: Submuscular transposition of the ulnar nerve at the elbow. In Rengachary SS, Wilkins RH (eds): Neurosurgical Operative Atlas. Park Ridge, IL, American Association of Neurological Surgeons, 1995, pp 225–233.
46. Mackinnon SE, Dellon AL: Experimental study of chronic nerve compression. Clinical implications. Hand Clin 2:639–650, 1986.
47. Mackinnon SE, Dellon AL: Surgery of the Peripheral Nerve. New York, Thieme, 1988.
48. Mackinnon SE, Dellon AL, Hudson AR, Hunter DA: A primate model for chronic nerve compression. J Reconstr Microsurg 1:185–194, 1985.
49. Mackinnon SE, Dellon AL, Hudson AR, Hunter DA: Chronic human nerve compression—a histological assessment. Neuropathol Appl Neurobiol 12:547–565, 1986.
50. Mackinnon SE, Novak CB: Clinial commentary: Pathogenesis of cumulative trauma disorder. J Hand Surg 19A:873–883, 1994.
51. Mackinnon SE, Novak CB: Evaluation of the patient with thoracic outlet syndrome. Semin Thorac Cardiovasc Surg 8:190–200, 1996.
52. Mackinnon SE, Novak CB: Repetitive strain in the workplace. J Hand Surg 22A:2–18, 1997.
53. Margolis W, Kraus JF: The prevalence of carpal tunnel syndrome symptoms in female supermarket checkers. J Occup Med 29:953–956, 1987.
54. Masear VR, Hays JM, Hyde AG: An industrial cause of carpal tunnel syndrome. J Hand Surg 11A:222–227, 1986.
55. McKenzie RA: The Cervical and Thoracic Spine. Waikanae, New Zealand, Spinal Publications, 1990.
56. McKenzie RA: Treat Your Own Neck. Waikanae, New Zealand, Spinal Publications, 1990.
57. Monsivais JJ, Bucher PA, Monsivais DB: Nonsurgically treated carpal tunnel syndrome in the manual worker. Plast Reconstr Surg 94:695–698, 1994.
58. Nilsson T, Hagberg M, Burstrom L, Kihlberg S: Impaired nerve conduction in the carpal tunnel of platers and truck assemblers exposed to hand-arm vibration. Scand J Work Environ Health 20:189–199, 1994.
59. Novak CB, Collins ED, Mackinnon SE: Outcome following conservative management of thoracic outlet syndrome. J Hand Surg 20A:542–548, 1995.
60. Novak CB, Lee GW, Mackinnon SE, Lay L: Provocative testing for cubital tunnel syndrome. J Hand Surg 19A:817–820, 1994.
61. Novak CB, Mackinnon SE, Brownlee R, Kelly L: Provocative sensory testing in carpal tunnel syndrome. J Hand Surg 17B:204–208, 1992.
62. Novak CB, Mackinnon SE, Patterson GA: Evaluation of patients with thoracic outlet syndrome. J Hand Surg 18A:292–299, 1993.
63. Novak CB, Mackinnon SE, Williams JI, Kelly L: Establishment of reliability in the evaluation of hand sensibility. Plast Reconstr Surg 92:311–322, 1993.
64. O'Brien JP, Mackinnon SE, MacLean AR, et al: A model of chronic nerve compression in the rat. Ann Plast Surg 19:430–435, 1987.
65. Osorio AM, Ames RG, Jones J, et al: Carpal tunnel syndrome among grocery store workers. Am J Ind Med 25:229–245, 1994.
66. Paley D, McMurtry RY: Median nerve compression test in carpal tunnel syndrome diagnosis reproduces signs and symptoms in affected wrist. Orthop Rev 14:41–45, 1985.
67. Pechan J, Julis I: The pressure measurement in the ulnar nerve. A contribution to the pathophysiology of the cubital tunnel syndrome. J Biomech 8:75–79, 1975.
68. Phalen GS: The carpal tunnel syndrome: Seventeen years experience in diagnosis and treatment of six hundred and fifty four hands. J Bone Joint Surg 48A:211–228, 1966.
69. Phalen GS: The carpal tunnel syndrome. Clinical evaluation of 598 hands. Clin Orthop 83:29–40, 1972.
70. Rayan GM, Jenson C, Duke J: Elbow flexion test in the normal population. J Hand Surg 17A:86–89, 1992.

71. Reid WD, Dechman G: Considerations when testing and training the respiratory muscles. Phys Ther 75:971–982, 1995.
72. Rempel DM, Manojlovic R, Levinsohn DG, et al: The effect of wearing a flexible wrist splint on carpal tunnel pressure during repetitive hand activity. J Hand Surg 19A:106–110, 1994.
73. Rojviroj S, Sirichativapee W, Kowsuwon W, et al: Pressures in the carpal tunnel: A comparison between patients with carpal tunnel syndrome and normal subjects. J Bone Joint Surg 72B:516–518, 1990.
74. Roos DB, Owens JC: Thoracic outlet syndrome. Arch Surg 93:71–74, 1966.
75. Sanders RJ, Haug CE: Thoracic Outlet Syndrome: A Common Sequela of Neck Injuries. Philadephia, JB Lippincott, 1991.
76. Schottland JR, Kirschberg GJ, Fillingim R, et al: Median nerve latencies in poultry processing workers: An approach to resolving the role of industrial "cumulative trauma" in the development of carpal tunnel syndrome. J Occup Med 33:627–631, 1991.
77. Silverstein BA, Fine LJ, Armstrong TJ: Occupation factors and carpal tunnel syndrome. Am J Ind Med 11:343–358, 1987.
78. Silverstein MA, Silverstein BA, Franklin GM: Evidence for work-related musculoskeletal disorders: A scientific counterargument. J Occup Environ Med 38:477–484, 1996.
79. Szabo RM, Chidley LK: Stress carpal tunnel pressures in patients with carpal tunnel syndrome and normal patients. J Hand Surg 14A:624–627, 1989.
80. Szabo RM, Gelberman RH, Dimick MP: Sensibility testing in patients with carpal tunnel syndrome. J Bone Joint Surg 66A:60–64, 1984.
81. Totten PA, Hunter JM: Therapeutic techniques to enhance nerve gliding in thoracic outlet syndrome and carpal tunnel syndrome. Hand Clin 7:505–520, 1991.
82. Travell JG, Simons DG: Myofascial Pain and Dysfunction. The Trigger Point Manual. Baltimore, Williams & Wilkins, 1983.
83. Upton ARM, McComas AJ: The double crush in nerve-entrapment syndromes. Lancet 2:359–362, 1973.
84. Urschel HC, Razzuk MA, Wood RE, et al: Objective diagnosis (ulnar nerve conduction velocity) and current therapy of the thoracic outlet syndrome. Ann Thorac Surg 12:608–620, 1971.
85. Weiland AJ: Repetitive strain injuries and cumulative trauma disorders. J Hand Surg 21A:337, 1996.
86. Weiss ND, Gordon L, Bloom T, et al: Position of the wrist associated with the lowest carpal-tunnel pressures: Implications for splint design. J Bone Joint Surg 77A:1695–1699, 1995.
87. White SG, Sahrmann SA: A movement balance system approach to management of musculoskeletal pain. In Grant R (ed): Clinics in Physical Therapy; Physical Therapy of the Cervical and Thoracic Spine. New York, Churchill Livingstone, 1994, pp 339–357.
88. Wilbourn AJ: The thoracic outlet syndrome is over-diagnosed. Arch Neurol 47:228–230, 1990.
89. Wilbourn AJ: Thoracic outlet syndromes—plea for conservatism. Neurosurg Clin North Am 2:235–245, 1991.
90. Wilbourn AJ, Lederman RJ: Evidence for conduction delay in thoracic outlet syndrome is challenged. N Engl J Med 310:1052–1053, 1984.
91. Williams TM, Mackinnon SE, Novak CB, et al: Verfication of the pressure provocative test in carpal tunnel syndrome. Ann Plast Surg 29:8–11, 1992.
92. Yiannikas C, Walsh JC: Somatosensory evoked responses in the diagnosis of thoracic outlet syndrome. J Neurol Neurosurg Psychiatry 46:234–240, 1983.

ALLARD E. DEMBE, ScD

THE CHANGING NATURE OF OFFICE WORK: EFFECTS ON REPETITIVE STRAIN INJURIES

From the Occupational and
  Environmental Health Program
University of Massachusetts
  Medical School
Worcester, Massachusetts

Reprint requests to:
Allard E. Dembe, ScD
Assistant Professor
Occupational and Environmental
  Health Program
Department of Family Medicine
  and Community Health
University of Massachusetts
  Medical School
55 Lake Avenue North
Worcester, MA 01655

The contemporary surge in the reporting of upper extremity repetitive strain injuries (RSIs) and occupational musculoskeletal disorders has coincided with the explosive growth of computers, video display terminals (VDTs), electronic keyboards, and other modern office technologies. Mounting epidemiologic evidence links the risk of contracting RSIs with the postures, motions, and forces involved in using these office tools. Some observers have concluded that RSIs are a recent phenomenon ushered into offices by the current revolution in computerized information systems.

Close examination of historical records, however, reveals a much more extended and complex history in which the continually changing interplay of office work, technology, medical knowledge, and social forces have combined in intricate ways during the past 150 years to spark recurring outbreaks of work-related musculoskeletal disorders among white-collar workers. This history reveals that RSIs among office workers cannot be understood simply as a by-product of particular mechanical contrivances or specific office tasks. Besides the obvious physical job characteristics, it is also necessary to consider the larger social and cultural context in which office work is performed, the nature of labor-management relations, the traits and background of the workforce, and prevailing medical and scientific approaches toward characterizing occupational disease. To help illustrate these points, this chapter gives a historical account of the changing nature of office work during the

19th and 20th centuries and its impact on the emergence of various forms of repetitive strain injuries.

OFFICE WORK IN THE NINETEENTH CENTURY

Although historians have traced the early origins of office work to recordkeeping practices used in ancient Egypt and China,[2,18] the growth of the modern office environment stems from changes in production methods that arose in Europe and the United States during the Industrial Revolution of the early 19th century. Tremendous changes in employment patterns occurred as a result of the vastly expanded scale of commerce, growth of banking and insurance industries, advances in railway transportation, and the introduction of a capitalist factory system. These changes produced a greatly expanded need for business-related correspondence, the maintenance of financial and legal records, and the speedy transmittal of information over great distances.

These developments led to an explosive growth in the hiring of scribes, copyists, bookkeepers, and clerks, who generally worked in areas physically separated from normal production operations. The emergence of this office workforce was initially most dramatic at banks, insurance companies, newspapers, government bureaus, postal and telegraph services, railway and steamship companies, and large factories. By 1850, more than 5% of workers in Great Britain, Germany, and the United States were engaged in white-collar employment.[11,25] These middle-class workers were mostly concentrated in large cities or the new suburbs that had been made possible by the establishment of commuter railways.

Prior to the 1880s, most office work was accomplished using pen and paper. Quill pens were commonplace, and mechanical pens began to be used after their introduction in the 1820s. Frequently, the writing tasks performed by workers were prolonged, detailed, and monotonous. Scribes, copyists, and bookkeepers often spent 10–12 hours per day writing manually.[37] From its inception, much office work was regimented and boring, performed in settings that were congested, uncomfortable, poorly lit, and inadequately ventilated.

Occupational maladies soon began to be reported. The most common affliction, writers' cramp, attracted considerable attention in the medical literature from its first description in 1830 through the end of the 19th century.[14] Also called scriveners' palsy, writers' cramp was considered by most medical authorities to be an occupational disease, associated primarily with the continual grasping and movement of a pen during the performance of clerical tasks. Interestingly, it occurred frequently in office workers but almost never among professional authors.[12,20,23] This led G. Vivan Poore and other leading researchers to conclude that the disorder was associated not only with the type of manual exertions performed but also with "the unwholesome life of a clerk who spends his days in a stuffy office in a crowded city."[33]

In what was perhaps one of the first examples of systematic ergonomics analysis and task redesign, medical experts identified specific risk factors for writers' cramp, including the force of pen prehension, the frequency of pen-stroke repetition, and the unyielding rigidity of steel pen tips.[14] Numerous improvements were suggested to alleviate the problem, including the use of rubber or cork sleeves, replacement of sharp steel tips with stub-end points, and the use of attachable penholders (Fig. 1).[12] After the introduction of mechanical typewriters in the 1880s, it was also commonly recommended that a typewriter should be used instead of manual writing to relieve the need for constant grasping.[14,20,33]

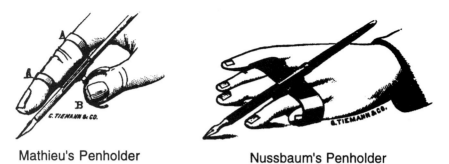

Mathieu's Penholder   **Nussbaum's Penholder**

FIGURE 1. Early ergonomics. (From Dana C: Textbook of Nervous Diseases. 3rd ed. New York, William Wood, 1894.)

Similar disorders of the hands and wrists began to appear in other groups of white-collar workers during the mid 19th century. Most notable was the epidemic of telegraphists' cramp that began to affect telegraph operators in Great Britain and the United States during the 1870s and 1880s. Like writers' cramp, this disease appeared in conjunction with profound economic changes and a massive surge of employment brought about by the introduction of new technologies and business practices. After the invention of the electronic telegraph in the late 1830s, telegraph communications expanded rapidly throughout Europe and America, and by 1870 tens of thousands of full-time telegraphists worked in railway and postal offices and in the offices of commercial telegraph companies, including Western Union in the United States and the Electric Telegraph Company in Britain.[14]

Telegraph work was also tedious, regimented, and performed for long hours without rest. It required constant motion of the thumb and index finger combined with the maintenance of a relatively static posture of the wrist and forearm (Fig. 2).[27] One investigator, Thomas Fulton, estimated in 1884 that a typical telegraphist made 30,000–40,000 finger contractions per hour, which is more than twice as many movements per hour as made by a contemporary typist.[19] By the 1890s, scores of telegraphists were reporting a variety of symptoms, including debilitating pain and numbness in the hand, wrist, and digits. Medical researchers linked the disorder to physical characteristics of the widely used Morse telegraph key as well as aspects of work organization, such as the failure to rotate workers between sending and receiving functions (to reduce periods of continuous key operation), excessive congestion

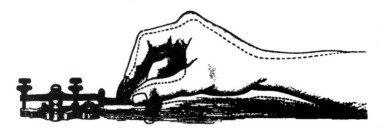

FIGURE 2. Normal position of the hand for telegraphing. (From Lloyd J: The Diseases of Occupations. In Stedman TL (ed): Twentieth Century Practice: An International Encyclopedia of Modern Medical Science by Leading Authorities of Europe and America. Vol 3. New York, William Wood Publishers, 1895, pp 456–496.)

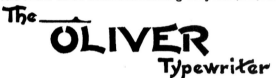

Railroad Telegraphers' Time-Saver

By using the speedy Oliver, you gain 50 per cent in time.

And you do this without the expenditure of extra physical or mental effort.

The Oliver meets the exacting demands of the railroad oper- ator's work.

Never gets "nervous prostra- tion," no matter how swift the pace.

The Oliver "works in a whisper"—in taking messages you catch every click of the sounder.

It "writes in sight"—you SEE just what you are doing.

It is a wonderfully versatile machine—instantly available for Wire Work Train Orders. Manifolding Way-Bills, etc., etc.

The OLIVER Typewriter

has many less parts than the old-style "mill" and is more compact and durable.

It runs smoothly, prints legibly, aligns accurately.

Special Terms to O. R. T. Men

You can OWN an Oliver Typewriter and pay for it by the month, the same as if you were renting it.

Let us tell you how easy it is to buy the Oliver on very small monthly payments. Ask for the Oliver Book.

Just mention in your letter that you are a member of the O. R. T. Address

The Oliver Typewriter Co., 169 Wabash Ave., Chicago, Ill.

FIGURE 3.   Advertisement from *The Railroad Telegrapher*, 1906.

in the operator's workspace, poor training and supervision, improper adjustment and spring resistance of the keys, and the nervous strain imposed on young workers as- signed to high-volume circuits.[20,27,31] Experts offered a variety of what are now called ergonomic solutions: armrests, redesign of the telegraph keys, job rotation, and, after 1885, expanded use of typewriters for receiving and transcribing messages (Fig. 3).[14]

Some commentators of the period believed that the high reporting of telegraphists' cramp in Great Britain benefited from the strength of the telegraphists' union and its campaigns for higher wages and better working conditions during the late 19th and early 20th centuries. Clerks, bookkeepers, and scribes suffering from writers' cramp in the 19th century were generally unorganized but shared with the telegraphists a middle-class status with relatively higher wages and social position than blue-collar factory laborers. In addition, through most of the 19th century, most white-collar office workers were men. The combination of a male, middle-class, literate, and politically well-positioned workforce may have made it easier for affected workers to have gotten their hand and wrist problems recognized as legitimate occupational disorders by physicians, employers, and government officials.

THE INTRODUCTION OF THE TYPEWRITER
AND FEMALE OFFICE WORKERS

Contemporary scholars have argued that the introduction of the mechanical typewriter, more than any other single technologic development, helped shape the modern office environment and the characteristics of its workforce.[2,3,13,34,40] The first typewriters—which appeared in the United States in the early 1870s—were relatively slow and difficult to operate, but improvements had been made by the late 1880s, and typewriters began to be widely accepted in office work. Because using a typewriter is faster than writing manually, companies could better respond to the growing demand for business correspondence that was resulting from a booming economy and the introduction of hierarchical corporate organizational structures in the late 19th century.[13] A new job category of "typist" had emerged, and large numbers of typists were being hired. By 1900, more than 100,000 typists were at work in the United States alone.[13,24,34,40]

In light of the well-documented incidence of hand/wrist RSIs among clerks and telegraphists and the need for typists to perform similar repetitive and manually intensive tasks, it would have been natural to expect that analogous RSI outbreaks would have occurred among typists. Surprisingly, few such health problems were reported. In speculating why epidemics of "typewriters' wrist" never materialized, many authorities of the time argued that typewriters were less biomechanically strenuous to use than steel pens or telegraph keys.[20,32,33,44] The simplicity and ease of operation of typewriters were extolled by Remington and other office machine companies eager to create and expand a market for their products.[9,13,25,36]

While typewriters may be inherently less dangerous than pens or telegraph keys, it is more likely that social and cultural factors involving the changing composition of the office workforce were chiefly responsible for the absence of a discernible incidence of RSIs among typists. With the advent of typewriters in the late 1880s, the demographics of the office workforce began to change dramatically. Before then, most clerks, scribes, and copyists had been male, middle-class, full-time employees. By contrast, after 1885 most typists were young women who worked for considerably lower wages than male clerks. A typical female office worker in the late 19th and early 20th century was unmarried and 17–24 years old. For many female office workers, employment constituted a temporary interval preceding marriage. The duration of their employment averaged 15–20 months.[11,13,25,34,36]

Employment of clerical workers in the United States swelled in 1880–1930, rising from 160,000 in 1880, to 737,000 in 1900, and to 4.0 million, or 8.2% of the workforce, in 1930.[34] Most of these new workers were women. Women represented 40% of all typists and stenographers in 1880, 76% in 1900, and more than 95% by 1930.[13,25] Women typists ordinarily could be hired for lower wages than male office workers with comparable education and skill levels. In 1902, male clerks in Boston earned about 50% higher weekly wages than women performing the same duties.[13,25,36]

At the time, some authorities justified the employment of female typists by claiming that women were physically and mentally better suited to typing than were men. One writer compared using a typewriter to piano-playing and concluded that it therefore fit better with women's "natural abilities."[2] Another claimed that the use of a typewriter keyboard was more appropriate for women than for men because men were handicapped by the "extremely large and strong fingers."[13] A 1913 article in *Scientific American* reported on a study that measured muscular sensibility with a "myo-esthesimeter," hand strength with a "Reginier-Cheron dynamometer," tactile sense with a "Weber compass," and auditory reaction time with a "d'Arsonval chronoscope;" the study found that women were especially well suited for typing because of their tactile and muscular sensibility, excellent memory for letters, and keen and sustained attention.[13]

Critics of employing women as typists countered that women were mentally, emotionally, or biologically unsuited for work in offices. The author of a 1920 article argued that women were poorly equipped for work in a business environment because they were "less strong, less agile, and less enduring under continued mental strain than men," a condition attributed by the author to the female menstrual cycle.[13] Some medical writers maintained that women's propensity to nervous exhaustion and neurasthenia made them ill-suited for office employment.[14,21,22,35]

Many contemporary historical studies have examined the forces responsible for the feminization of the office workforce that took place in Europe and the United States during the early 20th century.[2,3,20,11,13,25,34,36] While there is widespread agreement that the introduction of the typewriter was a pivotal development, most commentators believe that it facilitated, rather than caused, the entry of large numbers of women into clerical positions.[13,36] Primary reasons cited for the dramatic growth of female white-collar employment include women's higher rates of literacy (more women than men were graduated from high school), the lower prevailing wage rate for female versus male office workers, the decline of available domestic work for women, and the relatively better wages, shorter hours, and higher social status for women in office jobs compared to many other traditionally female occupations, including factory work, domestic service, and clerking in retail shops.[3,13,25,36]

The relatively brief tenure of most young women in office jobs also meant that employers could retain qualified workers without having to train them for advanced positions or pay them the higher wages that accompanied job experience and promotions. Some contemporary historians, notably Sharon Hartman Strom, cite this and other evidence to argue that the feminization of typing and other office work in the early 20th century reflected deep-seated societal gender discrimination that served to protect the privileged status of the entrenched male establishment.[36] According to this view, the relegation of women to dead-end, routinized typing jobs reinforced a prevailing image of women as docile, compliant, and unsuited to decision-making and other higher business functions.

Another factor commonly cited for shaping the modern office labor force is the rise of Taylorism and scientific management practices after 1910. Originally directed to factory work, the theories of Frederick Winslow Taylor were increasingly applied to rationalize typing, stenography, filing, and other office functions into discrete jobs performed in standardized ways under the direction of higher-grade supervisors.[18,36] Adopting the time-and-motion analysis techniques first developed by Frank Gilbreth for use in industrial settings, typing and other office jobs were differentiated and routinized, thus decreasing the information and control available to any particular clerical worker.[13,36] As women streamed into the office workforce, spurred by the labor shortages of World War I, they were shunted into increasingly mechanized de-skilled, and obsequious positions.

In this environment of low wages, poor job security, and little power, female typists and clerks would probably have been reluctant to seek medical treatment for hand and wrist problems. The typically brief tenure of their employment meant that disorders caused by the cumulative effect of repeated exposure to stressors were less likely to develop. If a disabling condition did arise, many typists would have been apt to end their employment and, consequently, fewer job injuries would have been reported. Those remaining on the job may have continued working despite pain or discomfort. The head of a large publishing company remarked in 1910 that "women are much to be preferred [for clerical work] for a number of reasons. They are capable and industrious, and, so far as my personal experience goes absolutely reliable . . . Men are troublesome. They complain about trifles that a woman wouldn't notice . . . The women come whether they have headaches or not."[13]

THE TELEPHONE INDUSTRY

Another new type of technology that drew large numbers of young women into white-collar employment during the early 20th century was the telephone. The use of telephones grew rapidly after their invention by Alexander Graham Bell and Elisha Gray in 1876, especially in the United States. By 1885, there were 140,000 subscribers and 800 exchanges in the U.S., more than twice as many as in the rest of the world combined.[38] By 1910, nearly 100,000 persons worked at telephone switchboards, and more than 90% of them were women (Table 1).[24,41] The economic forces that made women attractive as telephone operators were essentially as for other white-collar jobs: high labor demand, the need for literate workers, and comparatively low wages for women. As was the case for typists, employers lauded the employment of women in telephone work because "the work of successful telephone operating demanded just the particular dexterity, patience and forbearance possessed by the average woman in a degree superior to that of the opposite sex."[28] Telephone companies in the United States and most European nations hired only young single women and expected them to resign upon marriage. As a result, turnover at many exchanges exceeded 100% per year.[28]

In a typical telephone exchange of the early 20th century, dozens of telephone operators sat side-by-side on hard wooden chairs in front of long rows of switchboards, with supervisors walking behind. Discipline was rigid, and mistakes were not tolerated.[43] The normal workday was $8\frac{1}{2}$ hours, but overtime and weekend work were common. According to observations made by the U.S. Department of Labor Women's Bureau, a telephone operator was expected to "sit erect, keep her arms close to her body, her feet flat on the floor or on the foot rails, her eyes glued to the board, and have an answering plug in one hand to catch the next incoming signal."[41] Making the connections required constant high-speed movements of the arms and shoulders as the operators reached to insert and remove plugs from different circuits.

TABLE 1.   Employment of Telephone Operators in United States

	Total in United States	% Female
1900	15,327	80.0
1910	88,262	90.2
1920	178,379	93.8
1930	235,259	94.5
1940	197,062	94.6
1941–44	< 175,000	99.9

Most operators were required to complete or disconnect a circuit in no more than 3 seconds so that, during heavy periods, an operator would be expected to handle a load of up to 1200 calls per hour.[7]

The job was reported to have involved considerable physical and nervous strain. According to a government report published in 1907, "The element of strain is increased sometimes by the excessive height of the switchboard, which varies from 18 inches to 30, and occasionally to 36 inches where traffic is heavy and the maximum number of lines is admitted to the exchange. At the higher boards, a girl can only with difficulty reach the upper row of jacks, unless she stands or stretches in her chair, a motion which involves physical strain and causes delay."[7] Medical authorities considered the job particularly hazardous. Dr. Robert Dwyer, one of 26 physicians testifying at a Royal Commission hearing on telephone work in Ottawa, Canada, in 1907, declared that "four or five hours would be the maximum time I would consider for telephone girls on account of the extraordinary tension of most of the faculties that the operator is under." Operators working more than 5 hours continuously would deteriorate, claimed Dwyer, because "they break down nervously and have nervous children and it is a loss to the community."[7]

Despite the extensive movements of the arms, shoulders, and hands required in telephone work, reports of upper extremity RSIs were rare. More common were accounts of hearing loss and ear damage from loud "metallic" or "crackling" noises caused by lightning or other occasionally high-voltage discharges.[14] There were also numerous complaints of fatigue, often described as "a fagged-out feeling and tense nerves at the end of the day."[41] The issue of fatigue was used by telephone workers and labor advocates as a basis for arguing for a maximum 8-hour workday, which was a popular cause during the Progressive Era.[42] Unlike other female office workers, many telephone workers were politically assertive, belonging to the International Brotherhood of Electrical Workers (IBEW) and other trade unions. Highly publicized strikes by militant telephone operators, mostly in New England, took place in 1913, 1919, and 1923.[14,43]

Nevertheless, for most early 20th century female telephone operators, job status was precarious, job tenure brief, and wage rates low. Rather than receiving the strong support of national labor movement, their demands often threatened the job security and preferential wage rates of the male membership of the IBEW, and dissension within the union ensued.[43] Further friction was directed at the telephone operators by male telegraph workers, whose jobs were rapidly being eliminated through the growth of the telephone. The general social reaction against organized labor and progressive causes in the United States during the 1920s further weakened the telephone workers' position, as did the Great Depression of the 1930s. By 1940, the employment of telephone operators began to decline (see Table 1) as manual telephone exchanges were replaced by dial telephones and automatic circuitry.[4,28] Thus, it is perhaps not surprising that, despite documented job hazards and the concerns of medical authorities, there was never an appreciable incidence of hand/wrist RSIs reported among telephone operators or other female office workers during the first half of the 20th century.

DEVELOPMENTS AFTER WORLD WAR II

This situation changed dramatically in the late 1970s and early 1980s. The incidence of occupational carpal tunnel syndrome and hand/wrist RSIs began to grow. By the late 1980s, it had become the most frequently reported type of occupational illness in the United States. According the the U.S. Bureau of Labor Statistics

(BLS), 439,000 new cases of RSI were reported in 1996, representing 64% of all recorded occupational illnesses.[39] A BLS survey found that many RSIs occur among office workers, with 22% of cases of carpal tunnel syndrome attributable to typing and keyboard activities.[5]

Several studies have tried to identify factors responsible for the sudden increase in reports of RSI that took place in 1985–1995. Reasons frequently cited include higher production rates, the shift toward service and high-technology jobs, liberalized workers' compensation laws, and expanded medical awareness of the relationship between compensation laws, and expanded medical awareness of the relationship between occupational stressors and the risk of contracting RSIs.[6,14] Many authorities have pointed to the introduction of VDTs and other computer technologies as a primary cause of the contemporary RSI epidemic. This view is represented by the following passage by Vernon Mogensen:

> Prior to the VDT, office workers typically performed a variety of tasks in the course of a day's work, such as writing, typing, filing, taking dictation, making mathematical calculations, and writing correspondence. The mix of tasks, interspersed with pauses, helped to give the musculoskeletal system a break from repetitive strain. The incorporation of these functions in the computer eliminated the need to stop typing to change paper, make corrections, or perform a different task. The lack of spontaneous work breaks and the speeded-up pace of VDT work contribute to the repetitive motion strain that causes CTDs [cumulative trauma disorders].[29]

Ergonomists have implicated physical aspects of computer workstation layout and design, awkward hand/wrist postures maintained during computer use, and the frequency and force requirements of keyboard input with the chance of sustaining an RSI.[17,26,30] Other researchers have found evidence of an association between contracting RSIs and psychosocial characteristics of computer work, including monotonous tasks, high perceived workload, time pressure, low control on the job, and lack of social support.[1,26]

The historical evidence described in this chapter suggests that routinized work, time pressure, awkward postures, and uncomfortable workstations per se are not unique to office workers using computers but were also present earlier in the century. Moreover, hand and wrist disorders related to repetitive office work have been documented by medical authorities for more than 150 years. Therefore, why did the reporting of work-related RSIs suddenly skyrocket in the mid 1980s? The increased use of computers and their inherent physical hazards may indeed have been an important determinant. However, other considerations involving the social and political environment in which office work is performed might have played a role.

The groundwork for concern about RSIs among office workers had been established by the confluence of several key social developments in the 1970s. Especially important was the growth of environmentalism and the feminist movement during the early 1970s, both of which were inspired, in part, by the success of the civil rights advances of the 1960s. Growing concern about the effects of environmental pollution helped bring increasing political attention to the insidious dangers posed by chemicals and other noxious agents in communities and workplaces. Widespread public apprehension about the dangers of environmental illness helped spur the passage of the national Environmental Policy Act in 1969 and the Occupational Safety and Health Act in 1970.

As new technologies, particularly VDTs, began to appear in American offices during the early 1970s, pervasive public concern about environmental dangers helped bring attention to the potential health risks posed by these devices. Nowhere was this concern greater than in the newspaper industry, where many journalists had been alerted to the possibility of health risks by their coverage of stories about the environment. The rapid introduction of VDTs at newspapers in the early 1970s for word processing and editing represented a major change in the industry's working environment that alarmed and worried many journalists. Many workers complained about eye strain, headache, musculoskeletal pain, and dizziness resulting from prolonged use of VDTs. With the backing of major worker unions, especially The Newspaper Guild, concerns were raised about the dangers of nonionizing radiation emitted by the VDTs, reproductive hazards to VDT operators, and vision impairment.[28] Ergonomic issues surrounding workers' use of VDTs became a major issue in collective bargaining campaigns at several newspapers during the mid 1970s. Several government investigations were launched, including a study by the National Institute for Occupational Safety and Health (NIOSH) in 1979 documenting that VDT workers at three major newspapers in California experienced high levels of workplace stress, musculoskeletal ailments, numbness in their hands, and loss of strength in their arms.[28]

The VDT issue became a central component of labor actions in the 1970s and early 1980s, reflecting, in part, deep-seated tensions that existed between newspaper owners and their workers. Concerns about VDT safety were picked up by other unions and became a major ingredient in organizing campaigns and collective bargaining efforts. In 1979, a VDT coalition was formed by The Newspaper Guild, the Office and Professional Employees International Union, and seven other labor organizations. 9 to 5, The National Association of Working Women, took a leading role in educating female office workers about the safety and health hazards of VDT use.[28] At about the same time, labor unrest and union activism in other sectors, particularly the meat processing industry, helped to bring national attention to the growing epidemic of carpal tunnel syndrome and other RSIs among various groups of workers.[14]

The growing concern about health hazards of VDT use among office workers in the 1970s coincided with the emergence of a politically active feminist movement in the United States. Several influential feminist critiques of gender-based discrimination in medical practice were published during the 1970s.[8,16] These and other feminist writings attacked the long-standing medical practice of ascribing nonspecific complaints in females to psychogenic or hormonal causes rather than acknowledging them as legitimate organic conditions. As epidemiologic evidence began to accumulate in the late 1970s for an association between workplace stressors and RSIs, the feminist perspective was important in helping to get carpal tunnel syndrome reinterpreted as a potential occupational condition. The prevailing medical view since the influential work on the subject by Dr. George Phalen in the early 1950s held that it was merely a female problem related to hormones.[14]

At about the same time, changes were occurring in the nation's workers' compensation insurance system. The changes were stimulated, in part, by the 1972 report of the National Commission on State Workman's Compensation Laws, which recommended that states increase the benefits available to injured workers and make it easier for affected workers to obtain compensation for nontraumatic occupational illnesses. Well-publicized court decisions in California and Michigan in the late 1970s expanded workers' compensation statutes to cover cases that develop gradually from the cumulative effect of repeated small strains or traumas.[14] Under this new doctrine of "cumulative trauma," a nonspecific ailment in the back or hands could qualify as a work-related condition eligible for compensation, even if it did not result from a specific injury occurring at a particular place and time. As scientific and political concern about hand and wrist disorders accelerated during the early 1980s, the increased reporting of RSIs and cumulative trauma disorders of the hands and wrists by workers, attorneys, and physicians may have reflected their attempt to describe the conditions in terms that would facilitate their acceptance within the prevailing legal system.

CONCLUSIONS

While the introduction of computers into offices may have intensified the biomechanical demands imposed on white-collar workers, a full understanding of the growth of reported RSIs since 1985 requires an appreciation of associated social and political developments surrounding that technological change. These developments include: the public's apprehension about environmental health risks, labor activism that brought attention to the dangers of VDT use, a growing feminist movement that expanded the political clout of female office workers and helped legitimatize their medical complaints, and legal changes in the state workers' compensation system that liberalized eligibility requirements for the reporting of occupational illnesses and created a new category of cumulative trauma disorders.

This chapter illustrates the more general point that there is rarely a simple connection between the demands of a particular technology and the risk of occupational disease. The reasons that the advent of telegraphs and steel pens prompted epidemics of hand and wrist complaints but the invention of the typewriter and telephone did not, may have as much to do with the nature of the white-collar workforce and its economic and political circumstances as with the physical demands imposed by the instruments themselves. This is an important point for ergonomists, physicians, and technicians to keep in mind as they examine the biomechanical and psychosocial characteristics of office work and attempt to mitigate the resulting exposure to occupational disease.

REFERENCES

1. Amick BC III, Celentano DD: Human factors epidemiology: An integrated approach to the study of health issues in office work. In Cohen BGF (ed): Human Aspects in Office Automation. Amsterdam, Elsevier, 1984, pp 153–166.
2. Armour H: New Technology in the Office Environment. Hampshire, England, Gower, 1986.
3. Baker EF: Technology and Woman's Work. New York, Columbia University Press, 1964.
4. Best EL: The Change from Manual to Dial Operation in the Telephone Industry. Washington, DC, Government Printing Office, 1933.
5. BLS Releases Expanded CTD Numbers. CTD News 6(7):3, 1997.
6. Brogmus GE, Sorock GS, Webster BS: Recent trends in work-related cumulative trauma disorders of the upper extremities in the United States: An evaluation of possible reasons. J Occup Environ Med 38:401–411, 1996.
7. Butler EB: Women and the Trades: Pittsburgh, 1907–1908. Pittsburgh, University of Pittsburgh Press, 1984.
8. Corea G: The Hidden Malpractice: How American Medicine Treats Women as Patients and Professionals. New York, William Morrow, 1977.
9. Cortada JW: Before the Computer: IBM, NCR, Burroughs, and Remington Rand and the Industry They Created, 1865–1956. Princeton, NJ, Princeton University Press, 1993.
10. Crompton R, Jones G: White-Collar Proletariat. Philadelphia, Temple University Press, 1984.
11. Crozier M: The World of the Office Worker. Chicago, University of Chicago Press, 1965.
12. Dana C: Textbook of Nervous Diseases. 3rd ed. New York, William Wood, 1894.
13. Davies MW: Woman's Place Is at the Typewriter: Office Work and Office Workers 1870–1930. Philadelphia, Temple University Press, 1982.
14. Dembe AE: Occupation and Disease: How Social Factors Affect the Conception of Work-Related Disorders. New Haven, Yale University Press, 1996.
15. Dempsey MV: The Occupational Progress of Women, 1910 to 1930. Washington, DC, Government Printing Office, 1933.

16. Ehrenreich B, English D: Complaints and Disorders: The Sexual Politics of Sickness. Old Westbury, NY, Feminist Press, 1973.
17. Feuerstein M, Armstrong T, Hickey P, Lincoln A: Computer keyboard force and upper extremity symptoms. J Occup Environ Med 39:1144–1153, 1997.
18. Field J: The office: A historical perspective. In Christie B (ed): Human Factors of Information Technology in the Office. Chichester, England, Wiley & Sons, 1985, pp 57–72.
19. Fulton T: Telegraphists' cramp. Edinburgh Clin Pathol J 1(17):369–375, 1884.
20. Gowers W: A Manual of Diseases of the Nervous System. Philadelphia, Blakiston, 1888.
21. Haller J: Neurasthenia: The medical profession and the "new woman" of late nineteenth century. N Y State J Med 71:473–482, 1971.
22. Haller J, Haller R: The Physician and Sexuality in Victorian America. Urbana, IL, University of Illinois Press, 1974.
23. Hamilton A: Nervous Diseases—Their Description and Treatment. 2nd ed. Philadelphia, Henry C. Lea, 1881.
24. Hooks JM: Women's Occupations Through Seven Decades. Washington, DC, Government Printing Office, 1947.
25. Kocka J: White Collar Workers in America 1890–1940: A Social-Political History in International Perspective. London, Sage Publications, 1981.
26. Kuorinka I, Forcier L: Work-Related Musculoskeletal Disorders (WMSDs): A Reference Book for Prevention. London, Taylor & Francis, 1995.
27. Lloyd J: The Diseases of Occupations. In Stedman TL (ed): Twentieth Century Practice: An International Encyclopedia of Modern Medical Science by Leading Authorities of Europe and America. Vol 3. New York, William Wood Publishers, 1895, pp 456–496.
28. Maddox B: Women and the switchboard. In de Sola Pool I (ed): The Social Impact of the Telephone. Cambridge, MA, MIT Press, 1977, pp 262–279.
29. Mogensen VL: Office Politics: Computers, Labor, and the Fight for Safety and Health. New Brunswick, NJ, Rutgers University Press, 1996.
30. National Institute for Occupational Safety and Health: Musculoskeletal Disorders and Workplace Factors. Cincinnati, NIOSH, 1997, DHHS publication 97-141.
31. Onimus M: Le mal télégraphique ou crampe télégraphique. Gazette Médicale de Paris 4:175, 1875.
32. Osler W: The Principles and Practice of Medicine. New York, D. Appleton, 1892.
33. Poore GV: Nervous Affections of the Hand. London, Smith, Elder, 1897.
34. Rotella EJ: From Home to Office: U.S. Women at Work 1870–1930. Ann Arbor, MI, UMI Research Press, 1981.
35. Smith-Rosenberg C, Rosenberg C: The female animal: Medical and biological views of woman and her role in nineteenth-century America. In Caplan AL, Englehardt HT Jr, McCartney JJ (eds): Concepts of Health and Disease: Interdisciplinary Perspectives. Reading, MA, Addison-Wesley, 1981, pp 281–303.
36. Strom SH: Beyond the Typewriter: Gender, Class, and the Origins of Modern American Office Work, 1900–1930. Urbana, IL, University of Illinois Press, 1992.
37. Thackrah C: The Effects of Arts, Trades, and Professions on Health and Longevity. Canton, MA, Science History Publications (1985), 1832.
38. Tucker D: Electrical communications. In Williams T (ed): A History of Technology. Vol 3. Oxford, Clarendon Press, 1978, pp 1220–1267.
39. U.S. Bureau of Labor Statistics: Survey of Occupational Injuries and Illnesses 1996. Washington, DC, Government Printing Office, 1997.
40. U.S. Department of Labor: Women's Jobs. Washington, DC, Government Printing Office, 1940.
41. U.S. Department of Labor: The Woman Telephone Operator. Washington, DC, Government Printing Office, 1946.
42. Webster GW: A Physiological Basis for the Shorter Working Day for Women. Washington, DC, Government Printing Office, 1921.
43. Wertheimer BM: We Were There: The Story of Working Women in America. New York, Pantheon Books, 1977.
44. Wood H: Functional nervous diseases. In Pepper W (ed): A Textbook of the Theory and Practice of Medicine. Philadelphia, WB Saunders, 1893, pp 651–654.

TIM MORSE, PhD

SURVEILLANCE AND THE PROBLEMS OF ASSESSING OFFICE-RELATED INJURY

From the Ergonomic Technology
    Center
University of Connecticut Health
    Center
Farmington, Connecticut

Reprint requests to:
Tim Morse, PhD
Ergonomic Technology Center
University of Connecticut Health
    Center
263 Farmington Avenue
Farmington, CT 06030-6210

Assessing the magnitude of work-related musculoskeletal disorders (WMDs) in an office setting is a complex task. A distinct difference exists between passive surveillance, such as basing an estimate of a problem on voiced complaints or workers' compensation reports, and active surveillance, such as performing a symptoms survey. This underreporting may be the result of a variety of factors, including low severity of symptoms, fear of retaliation for reporting, avoidance of paperwork, and lack of knowledge of reporting procedures.[1]

Evidence shows that early reporting, in combination with ergonomic intervention and conservative medical management, may be the key to a successful prevention program. Yet, active surveillance programs cause concern because they by definition will initially increase the number of reports of WMDs. Some managers are concerned that false positive reports may arise from people who become caught up in the issue. A spike in reports is not appealing even to safety officers or medical departments, which may believe that active surveillance is the best way to proceed.

This chapter covers reported WMDs in the office environment, differences in estimates based on active surveillance, the benefits of early reporting programs, models for estimating costs for WMDs, potential psychosocial issues, and some tools for early reporting programs.

REPORTED WMD IN OFFICE WORKERS

Passive surveillance of the workplace, which can use Occupational Safety and Health Administration (OSHA) 200 forms or workers' compensation records, is frequently used in identifying problem areas to address in a workplace.

OSHA 200 forms are not required for employers with fewer than 10 employees or for employers in low-hazard industries, which include many office-worker settings.* However, some of these employers will be required to participate in the OSHA annual survey of injuries and illnesses. Workers' compensation records are a second common source of information for passive surveillance.

Definitions of what types of illness are recordable differ somewhat between these systems. OSHA requires all illnesses, including WMDs, to be recorded on OSHA 200 forms regardless of whether they result in lost time. WMDs are recorded under "Disorders Associated with Repeated Trauma," which includes tendinitis, carpal tunnel syndrome, other WMDs, and noise-induced hearing loss. The emergence of new symptoms needs to be recorded separately even if there was a prior recorded case, and cases need to be recorded even if preexisting conditions existed from a prior employer or home if there are new work exposures that cause or aggravate the condition. Illnesses need to be diagnosed to be recordable but not just by medical personnel if symptoms are believed to be work-related, e.g., several workers at the same job are complaining of the same symptoms.[3]

These illnesses should be evaluated both by looking at the raw numbers of WMDs (to identify the largest magnitude problems) as well as by rates per full-time employees (to identify pockets of problem areas with the highest individual risks). Rates may help to target scarce resources on high-risk areas. Incidence rates in the OSHA/BLS (Bureau of Labor Statistics) survey are calculated based on an exposure base of 100 full-time employees, who are assumed to work 200,000 hours per year (40 hours × 50 weeks). To calculate this for a firm, use the formula N/EH × 200,000, where N is the number of illnesses or lost workdays and EH is the total number of hours worked by all employees (or employees for a particular area or occupation being analyzed) for the calendar year.[6]

Workers' compensation records overlap considerably with the BLS system but have some distinctions, which will become more pronounced when the new OSHA recordkeeping system is implemented. While individual employers can usually obtain comprehensive records of all illnesses that were submitted to the insurer, the numbers typically submitted to the state workers' compensation commission include only the conditions that result in lost time or select duty. Some states require only reporting of conditions that result in lost time beyond the state's waiting period, which is typically 3 days. WMDs often do not result in immediate lost time; if time is lost later, the case may end up not being reported even though it should have been. Therefore, workers' compensation statistics are typically lower than the equivalent OSHA/BLS reports.

Frazier and Loomis found that North Carolina workers' compensation records show that only 0.9% of 851 WMD claims were listed as related to computers or office equipment.[8] However, a review by the author of 807 WMD 1996 Connecticut workers' compensation reports reveals that 30% of WMD reports with identified occupations were clerically related occupations and that 10.5% of descriptions of WMD specifically noted exposure to computers, mouse, or data entry.

In Australia, Rowe et al. found incidence rates of 0.17% and 0.14% before and after an ergonomic intervention for clerical workers using video display terminals.[12]

---

* Standard Industrial Code (SIC) numbers 52–89 are excluded, with the exception of SIC 52, 53, 54, 70, 75, 76, 79, and 80.

The mean number of days absent from work dropped from 33.3 days for 75% of the cases to 3.4 days for 20%, and days of restricted duty dropped from 91 to 32 days. Also in Australia, Hocking found a rate of 69 reported WMD cases per 1000 annually (n = 1,886) for telephone operators doing data work at Telecom Australia and 57 per 1,000 (n = 1,421) for clerical computer operators.[10]

The BLS national survey (using OSHA 200 definitions) found that disorders associated with repeated trauma, such as carpal tunnel syndrome and noise-induced hearing loss, accounted for 4% of the 6.2 million workplace injuries and illnesses and 64% of the 439,000 total illness cases. The 281,000 repeated trauma cases reported in 1996 was 9% lower than the corresponding 1995 figure of 308,000 and 15% lower than the record 1994 figure of 332,000.

ACTIVE SURVEILLANCE OF OFFICE WORKERS

Active surveillance of WMDs involves looking beyond reported cases by using symptom or risk surveys. Such surveys have been used extensively in investigations of problem workplaces by the National Institute for Occupational Safety and Health, researchers, unions, and safety departments. Some employers have begun early intervention projects in which they actively encourage workers to report WMD symptoms in an attempt to avoid the more disabling and expensive chronic conditions. Techniques include body mapping, in which an outline of a body is presented to workers so that they can mark the location and type of musculoskeletal symptoms; written and oral questionnaires; and toll-free telephone numbers to call for reporting symptoms.

Cherniack reviews several studies of office workers showing increased WMD levels.[5] Hess found an increased level of reported WMD in an office survey, which also was related to reported psychosocial stress levels.[9] Using a symptom survey, Burt et al. reported an annual period prevalence of 40% (n = 331) for office workers in a newspaper office.[4]

A population-based random-digit dialing survey of WMD was conducted by the University of Connecticut Health Center's ErgoCenter in 1996 (the CUSP survey, Connecticut Upper-extremity Surveillance Project). The survey identified workers who reported significant upper extremity symptoms that appeared to be work-related.[7a] The study allows the description of period prevalent cases that are not reported to workers' compensation; it is essentially an active surveillance system on a population basis. Of the 292 work-related cases, 15.4% were in clerical workers, 25.7% in professional or technical workers, and 11.6% in managers and administrators. This shows a relatively high level of office-related CTDs. Of all the workers with WMDs, 54.3% used a computer and 23.7% used a computer more than 4 hours a day. Overall, only 10.6% of WMD cases had filed for workers' compensation, indicating the magnitude of under-reporting in passive surveillance systems.[10a]

Active surveillance also can theoretically be used in relation to biologic monitoring of workers based on surface electromyographic measures of force output or other measures of musculoskeletal stress, but this is unlikely to be used outside of a research setting. Similarly, surveillance of intrinsic risk factors is possible and could include measurement or observation of potentially risky posture and keying styles. Pascarelli and Quilter include posture issues such as resting hands on the desk and leaning on elbows, keying styles such as clacking (heavy force), thumb or pinky extension, and tight grip on a mouse.[11] These risk factors have their basis in clinical experience and physical medicine theory and are just beginning to be systematically evaluated.

Active surveillance of workstation design is more common, frequently with checklists or videotaping to identify problems. While this is used in primary prevention through workplace surveys, such workstation evaluations are commonly a result of diagnosis of WMD or early symptom reports. The latter can be used in a sentinel event model for identifying groups of workers performing work similar to one who has been identified as having a WMD. The sentinel event model is beginning to be codified in emerging ergonomics standards. For example, the California law on ergonomics requires workstation evaluation and controls where more than one employee has been diagnosed by a physician as having a WMD and was "performing the same repetitive motion task, such as but not limited to word processing, assembly, or loading" (California Title 8, General Industry Safety Orders Section 5110, "Ergonomics").

EARLY REPORTING PROGRAMS

Many employers are using early reporting systems, including active systems as well as reducing impediments to reporting. Impediments can include perceived negative consequences of reporting or increased paperwork and red tape. Behavioral safety systems such as "safety bingo," in which workers are rewarded for having few or no reported injuries or illnesses, can also act as impediments to reporting. Such systems can encourage safer behavior but also result in incentives and social pressures from coworkers to not report injuries and illnesses.

Two early reporting systems at Connecticut-based insurers are described below. Both were initially focused on employees of the insurer rather than policyholders, but one has branched out into a service for insureds.

The first system represents an attempt at centralizing WMD identification and prevention for a corporation that has an extensive network of field offices. The system is focused on a centrally located, one-stop service through a toll-free telephone number that a symptomatic employee at any location can call. The call is received by a gatekeeper whose function is demographic intake and determination of whether it is a workers' compensation case. All musculoskeletal cases are referred by the gatekeeper to the nurses in the ergonomics group regardless of whether the symptoms are work-related. The ergonomics nurse may recommend a medical visit, but this is determined on an individual basis and may not happen initially. The nurse's role is to provide education to the worker, which can include making an over-the-phone illness categorization, risk factor identification, and help for implementing ergonomic changes at the workstation. If the nurse determines that the case is work-related, she will route it back to the gatekeeper for the workers' compensation intake. Equipment changes are carried out locally. If the initial phone consultation does not result in symptom reduction, a second phone consultation can be used. The nurse may suggest medical consultation or give more advice about workstation set-up, sometimes by mailing the worker a videotape of the workstation. If problems persist, a traditional job assessment is carried out locally by a consultant/ergonomist. The insurer has found this system to be quite effective in reducing injury costs.

The second active surveillance model was initiated after review found high surgery rates—and related costs—for WMD cases. In a collaborative project with the University of Connecticut Health Center's ErgoCenter, Travelers Insurance has encouraged internal claims representatives with upper extremity WMD symptoms to report the symptoms and to have medical evaluation and treatment at the division of occupational and environmental medicine clinic.[7] From November 1994 through Fall 1998, about 320 patients had been seen in this program. All patients are seen by an occupational physician, an occupational therapist, an ergonomist, and a hand surgeon if necessary. Parallel to the early report/conservative treatment arm, patients' workstations and work practices are reviewed onsite by a Traveler's ergonomist. Formal communication regarding diagnosis, treatment, and ergonomic intervention takes place between the University of Connecticut and Travelers for every patient. Intervention modalities include workstation redesign, strengthening exercises, conservative medical treatment that may include nonsteroidal antiinflammatory medications, identification of nonoccupational contributors, and, when necessary, surgery. About 3% of the workers have required surgical intervention, which represents an approximate 90% reduction from prior to inception of the project. The data to date demonstrate the effectiveness of this multipronged approach: a reduction of Travelers' workers' compensation costs by 78% over 2 years and a resulting award for insurance innovation from *Risk and Insurance*.

ESTIMATING COSTS

The goal of occupational health is primarily to prevent unnecessary suffering for affected workers. The loss of full use of the hands from WMDs can have a devastating impact on activities of daily living, work roles, and family roles. While many employers share that prioritization, one of the more compelling approaches to motivate employers to institute prevention programs is a cost justification.

Costs for WMDs fall into several levels. The first is workers' compensation costs, which are typically the easiest to obtain and the easiest to assess in terms of economic advantages of prevention. You can also estimate indirect costs to the employer from lost time and diminished productivity. Hidden costs of WMD include costs related to group health insurance, sick time, and disability from unreported claims. Quality improvement is another related aspect but is somewhat distinct from productivity. Finally, costs are borne by the disabled worker, family, or by society that are not considered in an employer's cost-benefit calculation but are important for the greater social good and for regulatory consideration.

Some economic approaches simply try to crunch many of the indirect costs into typical cost multipliers that can be added to workers' compensation costs. Other approaches involve costing out some or many of the additional factors.

Workers' compensation costs appear to be straightforward. An employer can obtain from the insurer a report of the number of WMD claims for the past few years, including payouts for the claims broken down into medical and lost-time expenses. Three considerations complicate this analysis, as follows:

1. Future costs of claims may not be taken into account or are represented by a set-aside by the insurer of estimated future costs. Make sure to take that into account. Otherwise, the cost per claim may appear to be declining each year while, in reality, the longer-term costs simply have not been added in for the more recent claims.

2. Claims often are misclassified as strains and sprains and do not show up as "repetitive" for cause; however, this may be less of a problem in office environments than in manufacturing, where there are more strains and sprains. Such misclassifications can be reduced by asking the insurer for all claims or for all claims that involve the hand, arms, shoulders, and neck and those classed as repetitive.

3. Except for large firms that are self-insured, potential savings from prevention will be buffered by factors based on (1) size of employer (smaller firms will have a smaller proportion of their basic rate modifiable based on experience) and (2) typically a 3-year averaging (the full gain of prevention will not be felt by the employer until there have been 3 years of reduced claims).

The workers' compensation data should be reviewed by area and occupation, looking at both overall numbers and rates. For example, you may want to look at the rates per 100 employees by occupation. If the workplace is relatively small, you may need to group several years of data to compile such a breakdown with reasonable reliability. Rates show where intervention can be the most efficient or where to start a longer-term set of interventions, such as whether to spend the first available funds for new workstations, chairs, or other devices.

If little data are available, a sentinel event model can be used that takes the reported cases as a marker of more unreported cases. This can start a process of active surveillance (symptom surveys or workstation surveys) for that type of worker or direct preventive interventions for all similar workers.

PSYCHOSOCIAL ISSUES

Psychosocial issues, as applied to work-related risk factors, are important in WMD rates, disability levels, and reporting behavior.[2,13] Psychosocial issues can act as:
- A primary risk factor in the development of WMD, e.g., affecting muscle tension and speed of work
- A secondary risk factor increasing the physical risks in a job
- A symptom intensifier
- An obstacle to early reporting and treatment
- A factor to increase disability levels and length of disability

Psychosocial issues need to be considered in several different aspects in this context. Risk factors can be actively surveyed and addressed in a primary prevention mode, as in surveys designed to assess stress levels and in interactive training designed to identify causes and solutions. Stress surveys that have been developed by several unions and researchers can be used. Stress levels also can be addressed on an individual patient basis, with a view toward reducing the negative effects of the stress in the individual through behavioral or other interventions; however, this approach is less satisfactory because it is moving away from primary prevention.

The disparity between employer and employee perceptions of WMD risk factors can itself be a risk factor. Warren found that the greater the disparity between the perceptions, the greater the level of WMD risk factors.[13] Employee perceptions of risk tend to be normally distributed across firms, but employer perceptions are noticeably skewed toward low problems or no problems. Thus, a surveillance program might pay attention to differences in perception of risks and attempt to sensitize managers to risks and communication problems if significant employer-employee differences exist.

Obstacles to early reporting can be addressed by the firm through active encouragement of reporting, but a firm also must address any potential confounding messages from other sources, i.e., productivity mandates, safety contests that encourage nonreporting, and paperwork aggravation. Preliminary analysis of the ErgoCenter's CUSP data found that some of the factors that are important in WMD reporting to workers' compensation include (1) the severity of the condition, including expected loss of work time, (2) a belief that a claim is important for future problems, (3) fear of employer's or coworkers' reactions, (4) discouragement by the employer for filing a claim, and (5) knowledge of filing a claim. In a study of physician reports of occupational diseases in Michigan, Biddle et al. found that women, employees of small firms, and individuals with carpal tunnel syndrome were more likely to file claims.[1] They hypothesize that workers in small firms are less likely to have other sources of wage replacement or medical care and therefore need workers' compensation more. In relation to early reporting schemes, these issues would indicate a need to reduce perceived fear of reporting, increase awareness of reporting mechanisms, and ensure that workers are aware of the need for reporting less serious conditions.

Return-to-work programs also relate to these issues. In office environments, finding light-duty tasks that avoid further stresses to arms and hands can be difficult. Filing, for example, often is thought of as light duty even though the pinch grip used can be stressful, particularly with tightly packed files. Psychosocial issues can intensify these problems. Other employees and managers may feel that they have to unfairly assume the injured worker's tasks, and this peer pressure can result in too early return to full work or to full disability from increased stress levels.

TOOLS FOR OFFICE SURVEILLANCE OF WMD

Several questionnaires and other tools have been developed for active surveillance of WMDs by both symptom surveillance and risk factor surveillance. Body mapping is a simple approach that graphically depicts symptoms and is generally effective in many populations, including workers with low literacy skills. The activity consists of putting dots or letters on a simple drawing of the human body, with notations or color coding showing symptoms such as pain, numbness/tingling, aching, burning, swelling, and stiffness. The body maps are compiled for an area or occupation, which together show the types of symptoms that appear to be the biggest problem. The clusters can be analyzed by body part, symptom type, or area and occupation. The completed diagrams can be compelling arguments for ergonomic interventions in workplaces in which problems are extensive.

OSHA's proposed ergonomic standard,* which was abandoned several years ago, contained useful checklists for risk factors in an office environment. One computer checklist was fairly comprehensive, and another was shorter but accounted for time spent on tasks, which is useful information.

Using Surveillance Data

Active surveillance data can be used in medical intervention/return-to-work programs and in secondary and primary prevention.

Early identification of WMDs allows for more effective medical management through the use of conservative treatment modalities such as medical management and physical and occupational therapy. Avoidance of surgery can result in lower disability levels as well as dramatically lower costs for treatment and lost time. Retraining of individuals with potentially problematic typing styles also may be effective.

Medical treatment needs to be coupled with reduction of risk factors in computer set-up to avoid recurrence or exacerbation of problems. Early reporting should be coupled with workstation assessment and intervention and can be even more effective if workstations with similar characteristics are modified before users develop even early symptoms.

Checklists and computer programs** can be used in surveys to identify problem workstations, either coupled with symptom surveys or separately. Modifications

---

* Ergoweb's website (www.ergoweb.com) posts the abandoned standard at www.ergoweb.com/pub/info/std/oshaopts.html. It can be downloaded free.

** ErgoEaser is a free software program from the U.S. Dept. of Energy that allows calculation of proper computer workstation set-up based on the size of the operator. It is available at nattie.eh.doe.gov/others/ergoeaser/download.html

should always be evaluated to ensure effectiveness, and evaluations can include a repeat symptom survey to determine if symptoms have decreased or increased after the modification.

REFERENCES

1. Biddle J, Roberts K, Rosenman KD, Welch EM: What percentage of workers with work-related illnesses receive workers' compensation benefits? J Occup Environ Med 40:325–331, 1998.
2. Bongers PM, de Winter CR, Kompier MAJ, Hildebrandt VH: Psychosocial factors at work and musculoskeletal disease. Scand J Environ Health 19:297–312, 1993.
3. Bureau of Labor Statistics: Recordkeeping Guidelines for Occupational Injuries and Illnesses. Washington, DC, U.S. Dept. of Labor, 1986.
4. Burt S, Hornung R, Fine LJ: Health Hazard Evaluation Report. Newsday, Inc., Melville, New York. Cincinnati, National Institute for Occupational Safety and Health, 1990, HETA-89-250-2046.
5. Cherniack MG: Epidemiology of occupational disorders of the upper extremity. Occup Med State Art Rev 11:513–530, 1996.
6. ConnOSHA: Occupational Injuries and Illnesses in Connecticut, 1995. Wethersfield, CT, Connecticut Dept. of Labor, 1997.
7. CTD News: Travelers take dose of own ergo medicine. 6(1):2–4, 1997.
7a. Dillon C, Warren N, Morse T, et al: The Connecticut Upper Extremity Disorder Surveillance Project (CUSP): Sample description, survey methods, incidence and prevalence. J Rheumatol (submitted).
8. Frazier LM, Loomis DP: Usefulness of North Carolina workers' compensation data for surveillance of cumulative trauma disorders. Appl Occup Environ Hyg 11:1125–1130, 1996.
9. Hess D: Employee perceived stress. Relationship to the development of repetitive strain injury symptoms. AAOHN J 45:116–123, 1997.
10. Hocking B: Epidemiological aspects of repetition strain injury in Telecom Australia. Med J Aust 147:218–222, 1987.
10a. Morse TF, Dillon C, Warren N, et al: The economic and social consequences of work-related musculoskeletal disorders: The Connecticut upper-extremity surveillance project (CUSP). Int J Occup Med Environ Health 4(4), 1998.
11. Pascarelli E, Quilter D: Repetitive Strain Injury: A Computer User's Guide. New York, Wiley, 1994.
12. Rowe S, Oxenburgh M, Douglas D: Repetition strain injury in Australian VDU users. In Knave B, Wideback P-G (eds): Work With Display Units '86: International Scientific Conference on Work with Display Units. Amsterdam, Elsevier Science Publishers, 1987, pp 38–41.
13. Warren N, Dillon C, Morse T, et al: Biomechanical, psychosocial, and organizational risk factors for WRMSD: Population-based estimates. J Occup Health Psychol (submitted).

RT GUN, MBBS, FAFOM (RACP)
PT JEZUKAITIS, MBBS, FAFOM (RACP)

RSI: A PERSPECTIVE FROM ITS BIRTHPLACE

From the Department of Public
  Health
University of Adelaide
Adelaide, South Australia

Reprint requests to:
RT Gun
Department of Public Health
University of Adelaide
Adelaide, SA 5005

Upper limb pain is common, and there have been several reports of clusters of upper limb disorders in manual occupations.[43] However, Australia in the 1980s experienced an epidemic of disabling upper limb disorders that was unusual in several respects. The epidemic occurred predominantly in clerical workers, mostly female and mostly keyboard operators, an occupational group that had not been recognized as being at risk. The condition was characterized by severe pain and was often accompanied by symptoms such as allodynia, paresthesia, and hyperesthesia.[13] Although the symptoms were unaccompanied by physical signs of localized inflammation or degeneration, the condition frequently gave rise to prolonged disability.

The condition was given official status in 1982 and given the title of repetitive strain injury (RSI). The mechanism was described by the National Health and Medical Research Council as follows: "the constant repetition of movements imposes a cumulative work load which can cause pain and weakness and impaired function of the muscles and other soft tissues."[45]

RSI was notably common in the public sector, where the rate of resulting disability was particularly high. In one government department, an investigation followed industrial action over RSI. Of a workforce of 122 data processing operators, 26% had required treatment for RSI, 18% had symptoms or signs but had not sought treatment, 38% had symptoms only, and 18% were symptom-free.[51]

RSI was almost absent in female clerical workers in the early 1980s. These workers then

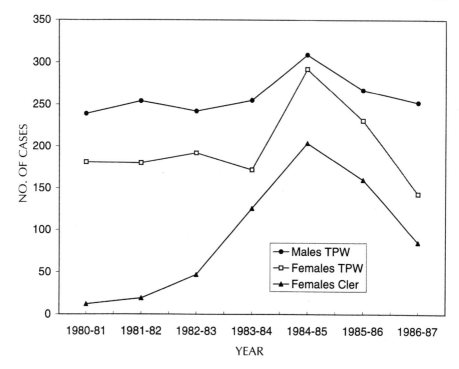

FIGURE 1. Diseases and injuries of the upper limb caused by repetitive movement, 1980–81 to 1986–87, by selected occupational categories, South Australia. TPW = tradespersons, process workers, laborers; Cler = clerical. (From Gun RT: The incidence and distribution of RSI in South Australia 1980–81 to 1986–87. Med J Aust 153:376–380, 1990; with permission.)

experienced an epidemic in which the incidence rose to a peak in 1984–85; it then declined, but to a level higher than that prior to the epidemic. Accompanying this white-collar epidemic was a smaller rise and fall in the incidence in female blue-collar workers, while in male blue-collar workers the incidence remained relatively constant. Figure 1 depicts the course of the epidemic.

The prolonged work incapacity, high cost, and loss of productivity of the epidemic provoked a vigorous official response. The newly formed National Occupational Health and Safety Commission (Worksafe Australia) prepared a Code of Practice for the prevention and management of RSI based on the assumption that the condition was caused by soft tissue injury or inflammation from repetitive manual work. Thus, the causes were assumed to be biomechanical, and an Australian Public Service Task Force Report, with little supporting evidence, suggested a number of pathophysiologic mechanisms: (1) reduced blood flow to muscles from tension leading to biochemical disturbance, (2) excess and unmet demand for synovial fluid, and (3) inflammatory effects from the breakdown of synovial fluid.[43] The concept of a physical injury or inflammation was given further status by the publication in the *Medical Journal of Australia* of a staging system that purported—without evidence—to be of prognostic value.[10] Stage 1 was said to be characterized by "aching and tiredness" of the affected limb, settling overnight or on days off work. It was said to persist for weeks or months but was reversible. In stage 2 there were persistent symptoms not settling at night, possibly accompanied by physical signs. Stage 3 was characterized by persistent symptoms at rest that "may last for months to years," and the authors reported that "advanced repetition injury may mean permanent incapacity for repetitive work."[10] Worksafe Australia publications endorsed the staging system, and its recommended preventive measures were based on a biomechanical explanation of RSI: setting of maximum keystroke rates, ergonomic workstation design, attention to posture, job rotation, and rest breaks.[56]

However, alternative views of RSI soon followed, leading to controversy in the Australian medical and sociological literature.

The title "repetitive strain injury" was itself criticized because it implied pathologic and etiologic attributes that had not been established. "Injury" implied tissue damage, and "repetition" and "strain" implied physical strain of tissues in causation, but convincing evidence of these assumptions was lacking. Indeed a characteristic of many cases of RSI was the lack of objective clinical signs of abnormality.[2] One of the alternative views was that the pain of RSI was due to a disturbance of sensory function rather than a soft tissue injury;[12] alternatively, RSI was interpreted as a form of epidemic hysteria or occupational neurosis (although this was not to imply psychiatric illness).[39] Medical practitioners whose uncritical acceptance of RSI as an injury that was caused by work were also blamed for contributing to the epidemic of psychogenic illness.[4] The title "repetitive strain injury" has now been acknowledged as inappropriate by regulatory and compensation bodies, and the title "occupational overuse syndrome" (OOS) is now preferred.

A common argument among those who denied the existence of RSI as a valid diagnosis was an apparent lack of awareness of the condition in other countries. The RSI epidemic was widely believed to be related to the rapid introduction of a new technology, such as visual display units (VDUs), which involved rapid keyboard activity and constrained postures. The fact that no such epidemic was reported in other countries also introducing this technology was construed as indicating that the condition was uniquely Australian.[2,18] Opponents of this view pointed to past outbreaks of occupationally related arm pain in Australia and elsewhere. A 1951 report of 544 patients with occupationally related tenosynovitis included 307 men from one factory in the United Kingdom.[52] The same report cited several previous clusters of tenosynovitis in a variety of occupations. In a comparative study of RSI in Australia and the United States, Hopkins described similar outbreaks in the meat processing industry in the U.S. and in the U.S. postal service.[31] In Australia, Ferguson had reported problems in telegraphists and process workers in the 1970s.[20]

While the occurrence of occupationally related arm pain and clusters of such cases is clearly not uniquely Australian, the 1980s epidemic of RSI in keyboard operators in Australia does appear to be unique (1) in its extraordinarily high incidence and severity, (2) in the absence of such epidemics in other countries, and (3) in that the disability was unaccompanied by physical signs.

To highlight the differences between this epidemic and other cases of upper limb disorders, a classification system was proposed. The better-defined clinical entities that have evidence of localized tissue injury or inflammation (e.g., tenosynovitis, carpal tunnel syndrome) were classified as type 1 RSI. Cases in which symptoms such as pain, paresthesia, or reduced grip strength occurred without evidence of localized disease were classified as type 2. Type 3 represented a combination of types 1 and 2.[38]

WHAT CAUSED THE RSI
EPIDEMIC OF THE 1980s?

The most important debate around the RSI epidemic was over its etiology.

Biomechanical Factors

Defining the syndrome as RSI implied that the condition was caused by mechanical factors in the workplace, and this view received official endorsement in the Code of Practice and other publications related to the prevention of RSI.

Although there is evidence for biomechanical causes of upper limb problems, little supporting evidence was provided to support such an explanation of the epidemic in clerical workers.

Most of the evidence relates to forceful tasks and high-velocity movements, with well-defined outcomes such as carpal tunnel syndrome, joint disease, tenosynovitis, rotator cuff disorders, and epicondylitis. For example, osteoarthritis occurs in the small joints of the hands of cotton pickers and in the knees and elbows in miners; upper limb disorders and carpal tunnel syndrome are prevalent in meat packers, process workers, and others with high exposures.[11,19,34]

In less strenuous tasks, this relationship has been more difficult to establish. Indeed, many studies of work-related musculoskeletal disorders often use office workers as the referent "unexposed" group. Studies frequently use symptoms rather than disease or disability as endpoints and have been vulnerable to inconsistencies in the evidence. In a cross-sectional study by Bergqvist on tension neck, as assessed by physiotherapists, an association was found between symptoms and the use of eyeglasses combined with VDU work for more than 20 hours per week, but no single factor related to repetitive work was found. Although increased risk was noted where there were limited opportunities for rest breaks, frequent overtime was associated with a reduced risk, implying a protective effect.[5] Lack of task variation and work deadlines were noted in a study of a newspaper workforce,[6] and more than 4–5 hours per day of VDU work was noted to be associated with a higher prevalence of neck symptoms.[33] Increasing risk of symptoms has been observed with increasing daily hours of VDU use.[47] On the other hand, in a study of a group of data entry workers, Ryan found that the difference in symptom prevalence was better described by workplace psychosocial factors than by time spent typing,[48] and in a study of VDU operators, Hales found that the number of keystrokes per day did not predict symptom prevalence.[27]

The concept of tissue overload may provide some biomechanical rationale for the RSI epidemic. Tissue injury to the musculoskeletal system can occur from an isolated forceful event but also from forces applied in a repeated manner. When under load, soft tissue structures such as muscles, tendons, and their attachments show physiologic characteristics such as lengthening, elasticity, and recoil. Such activity is essential in structural performance and in maintaining and increasing tissue strength. However, the capacity of soft tissues to adapt or repair may be exceeded so that repeated exposures alter soft tissue response characteristics. Thus, for example, tendon failure may result from repeated submaximal loads.[29]

Another mechanism for muscle injury may be related to inappropriate loading of muscle fibers. Static and dynamic muscle work may be optimally performed by different muscle fiber types (type 1 fibers)—slow twitch, glycolytic, sustained contraction—and type 2 fibers—fast twitch, short contraction duration, high strength), and the proportionate mix of fiber types may influence fatigability and contractile speed characteristics.[51] Abnormal physiologic effects from low-level stereotyped activity may occur by selective loading of inappropriate muscle fiber types or repeated loading of individual motor units. Changes in fiber ratio and muscle fiber histology may then follow from overuse. Thus, biopsies of the trapezius in regional myalgia patients have shown enlarged type 1 fibers and a reduced capillary-to-type 1 fiber ratio,[35] and similar changes have been reported in an Australian study of RSI patients.[15] Whether these changes are causal or as a consequence of disuse, neurogenic, or other factors is not clear.

The Telecom Studies

Notwithstanding this rationale, studies in Telecom Australia of workers with RSI provided strong evidence against a biomechanical explanation. In Telecom 3976 cases of RSI occurred during the 1980s (Fig. 2). From fewer than 20 cases in the first quarter of 1981, the epidemic peaked with more than 650 cases in the fourth quarter of 1984, declining to fewer than 100 cases in the first quarter of 1987. A number of interventions had been introduced over this time, including rest breaks and ergonomic furniture, but it was not certain that any or all of the interventions contributed to the decline in incidence from 1984. On the other hand, a number of findings in Telecom showed a distinct lack of any causal effect of the presumed biomechanical risk factors. The incidence of RSI was found to be no different in parttime than full-time workers, and no relation was found between the duration of employment and the prevalence of RSI. The apparent absence of any dose-response relationship suggested that the biomechanical factors were not causal.[30] More significantly, in a prevalence study comparing keyboard operators in different sections, Graham found that the areas of lower prevalence of RSI had poorer ergonomics but higher job satisfaction according to a questionnaire.[23] Comparison between different workgroups showed the incidence of RSI to be *inversely* related to the required keystroke rates.[30]

Psychosocial Factors

Thus, the studies conducted within Telecom indicate that biomechanical explanations for the RSI epidemic were implausible. However, studies by Graham, in Telecom, and Ryan suggest an important role of psychosocial factors.[23,48]

There is evidence of psychosocial stress in occupational groups affected by the RSI epidemic. Johansson et al. have demonstrated elevated urinary catecholamines and self-rated stress levels in workers whose tasks were repetitive, constrained, and machine-regulated, compared with workers whose tasks were less monotonous and more flexible.[32] In a study of VDU operators, Smith et al. showed elevated self-reported stress levels associated with workload, lack of control over activities, and boredom.[49]

Social influences also may have contributed significantly to the incidence of cases and the extent of disability. As the new keyboard technology was being widely introduced, there was increased attention to women's health issues, development of women's health movements, and involvement of unions directly and indirectly in the establishment of worker health centers. There also was greater activism in health and safety generally, with the establishment of an occupational health and safety unit of the Australian Council of Trade Unions and the election of a Labor government committed to empowerment of workers in health and safety matters.

Cross-sectional and longitudinal studies of neck and back disorders have shown an association between psychological variables and musculoskeletal symptoms. Correlations between distress and musculoskeletal symptoms have been noted in

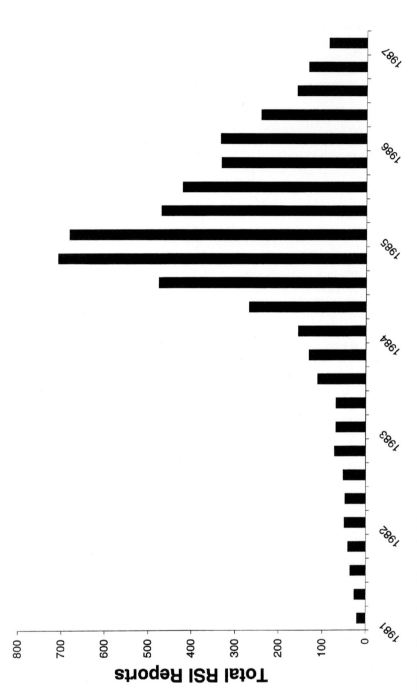

FIGURE 2. Cases of repetitive strain injury in Telecom by quarter, 1981–1987. (Adapted from Hocking B: Epidemiological aspects of "repetition strain injury" in Telecom Australia. Med J Aust 147:218–222, 1987; with permission.)

studies in which work has been mentally stressful and personally unsatisfying.[9] In a prospective study of white- and blue-collar workers, changes in clinical findings and musculoskeletal morbidity were observed to be better predicted by the quality of psychosocial, work content, and work control factors over a 10-year period than by physical loads. The association was stronger in white-collar workers.[36] Bigos has described a prospective relationship between psychosocial personal and workplace variables and the subsequent likelihood of being a back injury claimant.[7]

An Explanation From Gate-Control Theory

A substantial body of experimental and epidemiologic evidence now exists to justify a significant role of psychosocial factors in the RSI epidemic. The explanation is based on the gate-control theory of pain described by Wall and Melzack.[53] Pain perception previously was thought to be due to simple afferent impulses, transmitted mechanically from peripheral pain receptors through a system that was "hard-wired" in the nervous system. The gate-control theory has resulted in a number of new concepts, notably that of plasticity of the pain centers in the dorsal horn of the spinal cord, i.e., the ability of neurons to alter their structure and function in response to internal and external stimuli.[1]

Descending impulses relaying cortical influences to the pain centers in the spinal cord are likely to be of considerable significance. Extensive human and animal studies have shown the profound impact of environmental and social factors on central neurons, which respond to nociceptive afferent impulses and thus modify pain perceptions.[42] Thus, imputing a role for psychosocial influences does not imply that the symptoms are imagined. The gate-control mechanisms imply that such factors initiate a complex array of chemically mediated activities, resulting in functional changes in the dorsal horn and altered pain perception.

The concept of neuroplasticity also implicates collateral inhibitory and excitatory pathways in altering pain perception. One manifestation is that of wind-up, which is an increase in the number of action potentials elicited per stimulus in dorsal horn neurons, occurring in response to frequently repeated stimuli.[46] Nociceptive afferent barrages may thus have effects beyond the initial stimulus. In animals, post-injury sensory disturbances have resulted in continued pain; hyperalgesia and allodynia occurred with subsequent innocuous stimuli.[55]

The concepts of neuroplasticity may explain how social and environmental factors caused what would otherwise have been minor disorders to develop into the RSI epidemic. However, it does not explain what gave rise to the initial symptoms. Ferguson attributes the epidemic to a background of aching and discomfort—which are common in life and not necessarily caused by work—leading to widespread disability in the psychosocial climate of the 1980s.[21] Musculoskeletal pain and morbidity are prevalent conditions. The prevalence of chronic pain in the community has been estimated at 7–40%.[14] Fibromyalgia has been estimated to have a prevalence of 3–5% and to be six times more common in women than men.[54]

In an alternative explanation, Cohen et al. hypothesized that the normal ongoing afferent barrage of normal sensory data becomes misinterpreted. Their study was prompted by experience with more than 1000 RSI patients, typically with symptoms such as allodynia, hyperalgesia, and abnormal vasomotor and sudomotor phenomena. They suggested that increased receptivity and activity of the dorsal horn cells may be the result of constrained work postures and movements, which sensitized spinal neurons so that mechanoreceptive afferent information was processed as nociceptive.[13]

Iatrogenic Factors

Irrespective of the underlying causes of the RSI epidemic, it probably was worsened by a number of iatrogenic factors.

The recognition of the name RSI, and what it implies, by some of the medical profession no doubt led many workers with arm pain to identify their symptoms with a medical disorder. Labeling the disorder as a medical condition probably led to a greater willingness to make compensation claims and a greater likelihood that the claims would be accepted. This factor probably led to increased incapacity, which is prolonged by compensability.[22,24]

It is also highly probable that the staging system published in the *Medical Journal of Australia* contributed to the incidence and prolonged disability of RSI.[10] As Wright noted, this widely publicized staging system may have led many people with arm pain to believe that they had a potentially severe injury of which only stage 1 was reversible. Therefore, many workers with arm pain believed that failure to become a patient would risk loss of one's career and impairment of activities of daily living.[57]

The practice of some physicians in prescribing strict rest also may have aggravated the severity of the epidemic. Recent evidence supports views that overly prescribing inactivity or placing restrictions may lead to prolonged incapacity.[16,17,28,37,41,44]

REPETITIVE STRESS INJURIES IN THE 1990s

Contrary to popular belief, the incidence of occupational upper limb disorders has not declined in the 1990s. However, its distribution has changed. Table 1 shows the numbers of cases in South Australia from 1980–81 to 1994–95, based on statistics for workers' compensation diseases that resulted in the more than 5 consecutive days of lost working time.

The statistics cover three broad rubrics:

1. Mononeuritis. This category includes carpal tunnel syndrome, and this condition accounted for almost all cases in this category.

TABLE 1.   Repetitive Strain Injuries and Related Disorders, South Australia, 1980–1995

Year	Males	Females
1980–81	284	236
1981–82	339	276
1982–83	320	309
1983–84	357	396
1984–85	389	612
1985–86	370	508
1986–87	345	334
1987–88	*	*
1988–89	489	407
1989–90	618	467
1990–91	485	370
1991–92	479	400
1992–93	549	433
1993–94	614	507
1994–95	641	507

* Complete statistics unavailable for 1987–88

TABLE 2. Incidence Rates for Repetitive Strain Injuries and Related Disorders, South Australia, Mid 1980s to the Mid 1990s

Selected Occupational Categories (No. Cases/10,000 Person-Years)	1985–1986	1988–89 to 1990–91	1992–93 to 1994–95
Female clerical workers	25	9	11
Female tradespersons, laborers, etc.	106	70	76
Male tradespersons, laborers, etc.	23	48	44

2. Diseases of muscles and tendons and other soft tissues. Conditions characterized as OOS, which is the name given to conditions previously categorized as RSI, are placed in this category.

3. Cases that had been certified by the medical practitioner as injuries rather than diseases but were nevertheless attributed to repetitive movement. Only such cases affecting the upper limb were included.

In men, the number of cases overall have been consistently higher in the 1990s than in the 1980s; in women the numbers in the 1990s and in the latter half of the 1980s have been fairly similar.

Table 2 shows the incidence rate by broad occupational category. In men, who were not significantly affected by the RSI epidemic of the 1980s, the incidence in blue-collar workers rose in the early 1990s and has remained fairly constant. In female clerical workers, the incidence fell by one half in the latter 1980s and has remained low. In female blue-collar workers, who were to some extent affected in the epidemic, the incidence fell by one quarter in the early 1990s, and has since risen slightly. Thus, these soft tissue disorders are still common in the 1990s in female blue-collar workers and even more common in male blue-collar workers than during the 1980s.

Another important feature of these conditions in the 1990s is that medical practitioners usually assign diagnoses of conditions that are better-defined than RSI or OOs. Although OOS is recognized as a compensable condition by Australian compensation authorities, this title is rarely used by doctors. Table 3 shows the frequency of medical diagnoses made in a sample of 100 successive claims in 1994–95. Although comparable information is not available from the 1980s, cases of "type 2 RSI" appear to be few.*

Another feature is the increasing diagnosis of carpal tunnel syndrome—from 8% of all cases at the beginning of the period studied to 23% in 1994–95. This finding probably represents a greater use of nerve conduction studies in workers with upper limb problems than a true increase in incidence.

Table 4 shows the incidence of RSI by industry in the three periods from 1988–89 to 1990–91, after the epidemic in female clerical workers had subsided.

For men relatively high rates are found throughout the manufacturing sector, especially in food and beverages.

---

* Since 1991 diseases of soft tissue have been coded according to the mechanism of injury. On the basis of the data for mechanism of injury, only about half of the total claims are caused by repetitive movement, and most of the others are attributed to single events such as lifting or carrying. However, the nature of the reporting system leads to an underestimation of conditions caused by repetitive movement. In South Australia, the compensation claim form requires the doctor to nominate an occurrence (and the date of occurrence) that gave rise to the condition. Furthermore, workers are likely to perceive, correctly, that an injury at work is less likely to be challenged as work-related than a condition that had a gradual onset. The legislation makes it easier for a claim to succeed if it arose from an accident rather than as a disease process.

TABLE 3. Categories of Medical Diagnosis Accompanying 100 Successive Claims Categorized as Diseases of Soft Tissue, South Australia, 1994–95*

Condition	No.
Shoulder conditions (painful arc syndrome, rotator cuff disorder, tendonitis of shoulder, impingement syndrome)	32
Epicondylitis (medial or lateral)	24
Tendonitis, tenosynovitis, or soft tissue injury of wrist	16
Ganglion	5
De Quervain's tenosynovitis	2
Other	21

* Includes occupational overuse syndrome; excludes carpal tunnel syndrome

In women, the pattern is markedly different in two respects. First, the incidence is more variable in the manufacturing sector. The result of this finding is that the male-to-female incidence ratio varies substantially, suggesting that the difference is related to differences in the type of work to which men and women are assigned rather than to biologic factors.

The second is that in women workers the incidence is exceptionally high in a limited number of categories in the manufacturing sector—textiles, clothing and

TABLE 4. Incidence Rates of Repetitive Strain Injuries and Related Disorders by Gender, 1988–1991

Industry	Males*	Females*
Agriculture, forestry, fishing and hunting	61.9	81.4
Mining	15.5	11.1
Manufacturing		
Food, beverages and tobacco	75.2	105.6
Textiles, clothing and footwear	36.1	95.0
Wood and wood products	40.1	63.0
Paper, paper products, printing and publishing	13.2	63.4
Chemicals, petroleum and coal products	12.5	9.3
Nonmetallic mineral products	55.3	0
Basic metal products	56.6	63.9
Fabricated metal products	55.4	85.8
Transport equipment	51.2	139.9
Other machinery and equipment	30.8	113.9
Miscellaneous manufacturing	45.1	231.2
Total manufacturing	44.4	101.2
Electricity, gas and water	10.1	46.7
Construction	47.2	4.4
Wholesale and retail trade	10.6	13.2
Transport and storage	20.0	3.9
Communication	0	0
Finance, property and business services	4.6	11.7
Public administration and defense	9.9	9.2
Community Services		
Health	5.8	13.8
Education, museum and library services	2.1	5.9
Welfare and religious institutions	3.9	11.4
Other community services	11.9	5.2
Total community services	5.3	10.3
Recreation, personal and other services	7.9	11.7
Total	**22.8**	**20.9**

* Number of injuries/10,000 person-years

footwear, transport equipment, other machinery and equipment, and miscellaneous manufacturing. In miscellaneous manufacturing, the incidence rates have risen even further from the exceptionally high levels of the mid 1980s. The female production workers in these industries perform work that is repetitive; production bonuses are not uncommon, thus creating pressures for high work rates; and they have little job decision latitude, little control over their job environment, and few opportunities for promotion or career advancement. Thus, powerful risk factors exist for disabling musculoskeletal disorders. Yet, despite the evidence of the importance of psychosocial factors in the RSI epidemic of the 1980s, sociological evidence suggests that they are not of prime importance in the upper limb problems of the present time.

"Grateful Slaves"

Notwithstanding the fact that women in the manufacturing sector predominantly work in low-status jobs with little opportunity for promotion, considerable evidence suggests that these inequalities in the sexual division of labor are not manifested in differences in work satisfaction. On the contrary, several studies indicate that women are more satisfied with paid employment than men.

Some research in Australia shows that despite a greater degree of employment constraints reported by women, their overall job satisfaction was greater than for men, by a small but significant margin.[3] Other studies have similarly found that women report higher degrees of job satisfaction than men—even men with higher-status jobs—despite being concentrated in the lowest-grade, least-skilled jobs with the poorest benefits and prospects.[3,26] Baxter et al. concluded that the reason women are consistently more satisfied with their work than men lies in the way in which men and women experience employment constraints: "If men's occupational identity is closely bound outside the home, as the traditional image of the family breadwinner implies, constraints on men's opportunities to pursue paid work may have a more significant impact on men's satisfaction with work than is the case for women."[3]

In a report based on a series of group discussions and individual interviews with subjects ranging in age from 18–65, Mackay concluded: "For working mothers, paid work is often seen as a welcome break from the relentless demands of housekeeping and child-raising. Paid work is not 'leisure,' but it is certainly a welcome contrast with unpaid work at home."[40]

These findings, which Hakim has described as "the paradox of grateful slaves," compels caution in attributing musculoskeletal disabilities to psychosocial factors.[26] Although it is tempting to attribute the high incidence of these disorders to the repetitive and seemingly nonfulfilling tasks to which women are assigned, there is no justification for characterizing women workers, as a group, as alienated.

SYNTHESIZING THE EVIDENCE

The Australian experience is a tale of two RSIs—an endemic condition and an epidemic condition—which are different not only in occurrence and distribution but also in etiology.

The RSI epidemic of the 1980s was not caused by injury or inflammation but was a pain disorder. It affected a large number of workers, mostly female and mostly in an occupational category that was largely unaffected in countries other than Australia. The lack of response to conventional medical treatment, its severity (both in terms of days lost and functional impairment), and the common accompaniments of features such as allodynia, numbness, and reflex sympathetic dystrophy, suggest that this epidemic was qualitatively different than the current endemic conditions. Most importantly, the demonstrated *inverse* association of the occurrence of RSI in keyboard operators with presumed risk factors suggests that the causal factors were not primarily biomechanical. The decline in incidence of RSIs in the late 1980s followed a number of interventions aimed at alleged biomechanical causes. However, because none of the interventions were introduced as controlled trials, whether they were responsible for the decline of the epidemic was not determined. Other possible reasons for the decline were (1) a placebo effect, i.e., a nonspecific behavioral or psychological effect induced by the intervention irrespective of its content, (2) employees becoming reluctant to report the condition for fear of discrimination, or (3) a selection effect, i.e., all those at risk have either already developed the condition or have transferred to occupations with less risk. In the absence of evidence for a biomechanical cause for the epidemic, the most important influences appear to have been the unique social circumstances of the time. Thus, upper limb pains, common in life but usually transitory and nondisabling, led to a severe epidemic. However, attributing the epidemic to psychosocial factors is not to imply that the symptoms were imaginary; current theories of pain mechanisms confer a major role of situational factors in pain perception. The severity of the disability was probably aggravated by inappropriate labeling by the medical profession as an injury caused by repetitive motion, leading to misapprehension by patients as to the likelihood of prolonged disability. The perception of the condition as an injury or inflammatory condition also led to inappropriate prescription of rest, further aggravating the incapacity.

In contrast, the endemic problem of occupational upper limb disorders has not declined in the 1990s. Rather than being a single condition, a range of well-defined upper limb disorders exists that occurs mostly in the blue-collar workforce. Unlike the epidemic condition, these disorders are not unique to Australia.

The incidence of upper limb disorders varies between industries by two orders of magnitude. The highest incidence rates, by far, are found in the female blue-collar workforce engaged in production-line work in the manufacturing sector. This is no doubt a manifestation of the common observation that the repetitive, relatively unskilled tasks in such industries are overwhelmingly assigned to women. What is it about these jobs that causes upper limb disorders? Is it the repetitive physical demands of the work, or is it the psychosocial influences of being engaged in work situations that engender feelings of boredom, powerlessness, and alienation? The fact that women report higher degrees of job satisfaction than men suggests that the prime causal factors of upper limb disorders lie in the physical demands of repetitive work.

IMPLICATIONS FOR MANAGEMENT

The upper limb disorders described in the literature from many countries are different in many respects than the condition described as RSI that occurred in Australia in the 1980s. Accordingly, the biomechanical factors primarily responsible for the endemic problem of occupational upper limb disorders fail to explain the RSI epidemic of the 1980s. Conversely, the unique social causes of the Australian epidemic of the 1980s should not be used as a basis for inferences on the causes and management of occupational upper limb disorders occurring since then.

Analysis of incident cases of occupational upper limb disorders in recent years suggests that they are not homogenous. Rather, they include a range of well-defined clinical disorders, including rotator cuff injury, humeral epicondylitis, and carpal tunnel syndrome. The first aim in management should be to establish a specific diagnosis and institute appropriate medical treatment.

The insight provided by sociological research suggests that, when addressing the occupational causes, attention should be primarily focused on the physical requirements of the task, such as the issues of machine-pacing, posture, ergonomic tool design, and incentives to high work rates. The likelihood that such disorders can be prevented by ergonomic interventions is a cause for optimism: had the evidence suggested that the psychological and social environment was the prime cause, no remedy would seem feasible short of social revolution.

However, psychosocial influences should not be ignored. As with all medical disorders, social and environmental factors influence pain perception. Ergonomic evaluation should not only address biomechanical risk factors but, also, issues such as job satisfaction, supervisory support or conflict, and the need for workers to have a measure of control over their work environment and work methods. Stressors from outside the workplace may also need to be addressed.

One of the common mistakes of the RSI epidemic was the prescription of rest. Chronic pain, not associated with injury or inflammation, is not responsive to rest. The concept in the 1980s that RSI was an injury led to the erroneous interpretation of pain as an injury response to be managed by rest, splinting, and prolonged time away from work.[12] However, even for the better-defined endemic disorders, prolonged rest is generally inadvisable. Physical activity is usually sound rehabilitation practice. Experience from the management of back disorders provides epidemiologic, physiologic, and experimental evidence that return to work has some therapeutic effect, whereas prolonged inactivity is likely to increase the degree of disability.[16,17,28,37,41,44]

ACKNOWLEDGMENT

The authors gratefully acknowledge the assistance of the Research and Advisory Unit of the WorkCover Corporation of South Australia and of Donna Dias in particular, in compiling workers' compensation statistics for South Australia.

REFERENCES

1. Arnstein PM: The neuroplastic phenomenon: A physiologic link between chronic pain and learning. J Neurosci Nurs 29:179–186, 1997.
2. Awerbuch M: RSI, or "Kangaroo paw." Med J Aust 142:237–238, 1985.
3. Baxter J, Lynch-Blosse M, Western J: Gender differences in work satisfaction. Aust J Soc Issues 31:291–309, 1996.
4. Bell DS: "Repetition strain injury": An iatrogenic epidemic of simulated injury. Med J Aust 151:280–283, 1989.
5. Bergqvist U, Wolgast E, Nilsson B, et al: The influence of VDT work on musculoskeletal disorders. Ergonomics 38:754–762, 1995.
6. Bernard B, Sauter S, Fine LJ, et al: Job task and psychosocial risk factors for work-related musculoskeletal disorders among newspaper employees. Scand J Work Environ Health 20:417–426, 1994.
7. Bigos SJ, Battie MC, Spengler DM, et al: A longitudinal prospective study of industrial back injury reporting. Clin Orthop 279:21–34, 1992.
8. Bokemeier JL, Lacy WB: Job values, rewards, and work conditions as factors in job satisfaction among men and women. Sociolog Q 28:189–204, 1986.
9. Bongers PM, de Winter CR, Kompier MAJ, Hildebrandt VH: Psychosocial factors at work and musculoskeletal disease. Scand J Work Environ Health 19:297–312, 1993.
10. Browne CD, Nolan BM, Faithfull DK: Occupational repetition strain injuries: Guidelines for diagnosis and management. Med J Aust 140:329–332, 1984.
11. Cherniack MG: Upper extremity disorders. In Rosenstock L, Cullen MR (eds): Textbook of Clinical Occupational and Environmental Medicine. Philadelphia, WB Saunders, 1994, pp 376–388.

12. Cleland LG: "RSI": A model of social iatrogenesis. Med J Aust 147:236–239, 1987.
13. Cohen ML, Arroyo JF, Champion GD, Browne CD: In search of the pathogenesis of refractory cervi-cobrachial syndrome. A deconstruction of the RSI phenomenon. Med J Aust 156:432–436, 1992.
14. Crombie IK, Davies HTO, Macrae WA: The epidemiology of chronic pain: Time for new directions. Pain 57:1–3, 1994.
15. Dennett X, Fry HJH: Overuse syndrome: A muscle biopsy study. Lancet 859:905–908, 1988.
16. Deyo RA, Diehl AK, Rosenthal M: How many days of bed rest for acute low back pain? A random-ized clinical trial. N Engl J Med 315:1064–1070, 1986.
17. Deyo RA: Nonsurgical care of low back pain. Neurosurg Clin North Am 2:851–862, 1991.
18. Dodd P: Occupational pain syndromes [letter]. Med J Aust 144:501, 1986.
19. Edril M, Dickerson OB, Glackin E: Cumulative trauma disorders of the upper extremity. In Zenz C (ed): Occupational Medicine. St. Louis, Mosby, 1994, pp 48–63.
20. Ferguson D: Repetition injuries in process workers. Med J Aust 2:408–412, 1971.
21. Ferguson DA: "RSI": Putting the epidemic to rest. Med J Aust 147:213–214, 1987.
22. Filan SL: The effect of workers' or third party compensation on return to work after hand surgery. Med J Aust 16:80–82, 1996.
23. Graham G: Job satisfaction and repetition strain injury [dissertation]. Adelaide, Australia, SA Institute of Technology, 1985.
24. Greenough CG, Fraser RD: The effects of compensation on recovery from low-back injury. Spine 14:947–955, 1989.
25. Gun RT: The incidence and distribution of RSI in South Australia 1980–81 to 1986–87. Med J Aust 153:376–380, 1990.
26. Hakim C: Grateful slaves and self-made women: Fact and fantasy in women's work orientations. Eur Soc Rev 7:101–121, 1991.
27. Hales TR, Sauter SL, Peterson MR, et al: Musculoskeletal disorders among visual display terminal users in a telecommunications company. Ergonomics 37:1603–1621, 1944.
28. Hall H, McIntosh G, Melles T, et al: Effect of discharge recommendations on outcomes. Spine 19:2033–2037, 1994.
29. Hart DA, Frank CB, Bray RC: Inflammatory processes in overuse syndromes: Potential role of neu-rogenic mechanisms in tendons and ligaments. In Gordon SL, et al (eds): Repetitive Motion Disorders of the Upper Extremity. Rosemont, IL, American Academy of Orthopaedic Surgeons, 1995, pp 247–262.
30. Hocking B: Epidemiological aspects of "repetition strain injury" in Telecom Australia. Med J Aust 147:218–222, 1987.
31. Hopkins A: The social recognition of repetition strain injuries: An Australian/American comparison. Soc Sci Med 30:365–372, 1990.
32. Johansson G, Aronsson G, Lindstrom BO: Social and neuroendocrine stress reactions in highly mechanised work. Ergonomics 21:583–599, 1978.
33. Kamwendo K, Linton SJ, Moritz U: Neck and shoulder disorders in medical secretaries. Part 1. Pain prevalence and risk factors. Scand J Rehabil Med 23:127–133, 1991.
34. Kuorinka I, Forcina L (eds): Work-Related Musculoskeletal Disorders (WMSDS): A Reference Book for Prevention. London, Taylor and Francis, 1995, pp 3–14.
35. Larrson SE, Bodeman I, Henrikson KG, Oberg PA: Chronic trapezius myalgia: Morphology and blood flow studied in 17 patients. Acta Orthop Scand 61:394–398, 1990.
36. Leino PI, Hanninen V: Psychosocial factors at work in relation to back and limb disorders. Scand J Work Environ Health 21:134–142, 1995.
37. Lindstrom I, Ohlund C, Eek C, et al: The effect of graded activity on patients with subacute low back pain: A randomized prospective clinical study with an operant-conditioning behavioral approach. Phys Ther 72:279–290, 1992.
38. Littlejohn GO, Miller MH: Repetitive strain injury: Divide and conquer. Aust Fam Physician 15:409–413, 1986.
39. Lucire Y: Neurosis in the workplace. Med J Aust 145:323–326, 1986.
40. Mackay H: Work and Leisure: The Mackay Report. Lindfield, Australia, Mackay Research, 1994.
41. Malmivaara A: Evidence-based intervention for musculoskeletal disorders. Scand J Work Environ Health 23:161–163, 1997.
42. McGrath PA: Psychological aspects of pain perception. Arch Oral Biol 39(suppl):55S–62S, 1994.
43. Mullaly J, Grigg L: RSI: Integrating the major theories. Aust J Psychol 40:19–33, 1988.
44. Nachemson A: Work for all. For those with low back pain as well. Clin Orthop 179:77–85, 1983.
45. National Health and Medical Research Council: Approved Occupational Health Guide: Repetition Strain Injuries. Canberra, Australia, AGPS, 1982.
46. Pockett S: Spinal cord synaptic plasticity and chronic pain. Anesth Analg 80:173–179, 1995.

47. Rossignol AM, Morse EP, Summers VM, et al: Video display terminal use and reported health symptoms among Massachusetts clerical workers. J Occup Med 29:112–118, 1987.
48. Ryan GA, Bampton M: Comparison of data process operators with and without upper limb symptoms. Community Health Studies 12:63–68, 1988.
49. Smith MJ, Cohen BGF, Stammerjohn LW: An investigation of health complaints and job stress in video display operations. Hum Factors 23:387–400, 1981.
50. Taylor R, Pitcher M: Medical and ergonomic aspects of an industrial dispute concerning occupation-related conditions in data process operators. Community Health Studies 8:172–180, 1984.
51. Tesch P, Karlsson J: Isometric strength performance and muscle fibre distribution in man. Acta Physiol Scand 103:47, 1978.
52. Thompson AR, Plewes LW, Shaw EG: Peritendinitis crepitans and simple tenosynovitis: A clinical study of 544 cases in industry. Br J Ind Med 8:150–160, 1951.
53. Wall PD, Melzack RD (eds): Textbook of Pain. 3rd ed. Edinburgh, Churchill Livingstone, 1994.
54. Wolfe F, Ross K, Anderson J, et al: The prevalence and characteristics of fibromyalgia in the general population. Arthritis Rheum 38:19–28, 1995.
55. Woolf CJ: Evidence for a central component of post-injury pain sensitivity. Nature 306:686–688, 1983.
56. Worksafe Australia: RSI Training Package. Canberra, Australia, AGPS, 1986.
57. Wright GD: The failure of the "RSI" concept. Med J Aust 147:233–236, 1987.

BENJAMIN C. AMICK III, PHD
NAOMI G. SWANSON, PHD
HONG CHANG, PHD

OFFICE TECHNOLOGY AND MUSCULOSKELETAL DISORDERS: BUILDING AN ECOLOGICAL MODEL

From The Health Institute
New England Medical Center
Boston, Massachusetts (BCA, HC)
and
Division of Behavioral and
 Biomedical Sciences
National Institute for Occupational
 Safety and Health
Cincinnati, Ohio (NGS)

Reprint requests to:
Benjamin C. Amick III, PhD
The Health Institute
New England Medical Center
750 Washington Street
Box 345
Boston, MA 02111

The views expressed here are
those of the authors and not
necessarily those of the National
Institute for Occupational Safety
and Health.

Just as a shift from infectious to chronic disease epidemiology required new approaches for understanding the origins and patterns of disease, so too will we need to develop new ways of understanding the origins and patterns of illnesses and diseases produced by changes in technology from a human-mediated work process to a computer-mediated work process.[1]

There are no accurate statistics on the number of workers in the United States who routinely use computers in their jobs. Estimates of the number of people engaged in computer-mediated work also are difficult to determine. However, based on the number of workers in occupations known to use computers to some degree, a conservative estimate is that about half of the 120 million workers in the U.S. are now spending some time during the workday at a computer keyboard. With the continued rapid expansion of computer technology to all sectors of the economy, the numbers will only increase.

The effects of the physical aspects of the computer work environment on worker health have long been a concern; studies since the 1970s have indicated a link between ergonomic aspects of the work environment and musculoskeletal and other problems.[8,16,21,25,26,30] Although this research has prompted significant improvements in the design of office equipment and environments, musculoskeletal problems among computer users are still common. Thus, attention has increasingly turned to other occupational risk factors, namely work organization factors, which may, in conjunction with physical risk factors, play a role in the etiology of musculoskeletal disorders. Work organization is defined here as the way in which work is structured and managed, and it encompasses factors such as job design, the scheduling of work, interpersonal aspects of work, career issues, management practices, and organizational characteristics.[24] In this definition, work organization includes what have more commonly been called psychosocial factors or job stressors (e.g., job content factors such as skill usage and control; interpersonal relationships).

There is uncertainty regarding the ways in which work organization may be etiologically linked with musculoskeletal disorders. Models proposing a number of potential pathways have been developed but largely remain untested.[7,31-33,35] The ecological model of Sauter and Swanson will guide the analyses reported in this chapter.[32]

AN ECOLOGICAL MODEL OF MUSCULOSKELETAL DISORDERS IN OFFICE WORK

Although this ecological model was developed with office work and musculoskeletal disorders as the primary foci, it is a holistic approach that is applicable to other types of work environments and health outcomes. The model suggests various ways in which work organization and physical factors may act singly or in concert to result in musculoskeletal symptoms and disorders (Fig. 1). The major pathways include the following:

- Physical demands imposed by the job may lead to biomechanical strain and subsequent musculoskeletal outcomes.
- Changes in the way that work is organized (e.g., scheduling, job demands) can change the physical demands of the job, leading to musculoskeletal outcomes.
- Changes in work organization may create stress, which may result in increased biomechanical strain (e.g., increases in muscle tension) and an increased risk of musculoskeletal problems.

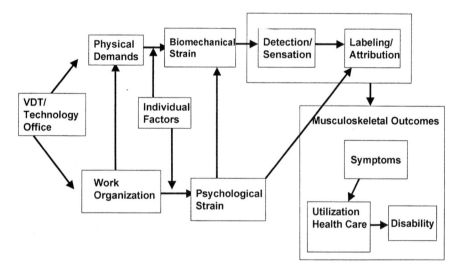

FIGURE 1. Model describing the paths from office technology to musculoskeletal outcomes. (Adapted from Sauter SL, Swanson NG: An ecological model of musculoskeletal disorders in office work. In Moon S, Sauter SL (eds): Beyond Biomechanics: Psychosocial Aspects of Musculoskeletal Disorders in Office Work. London, Taylor & Francis, 1996, pp 3–21.)

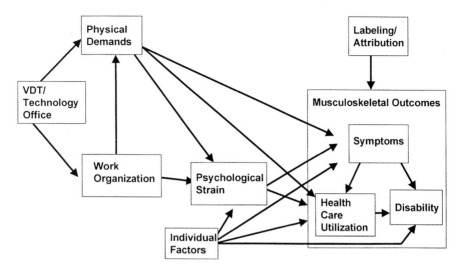

FIGURE 2. Modified model describing the analytic paths from office technology to musculoskeletal outcomes.

• Work organization factors may create psychological strain, which in turn may affect the detection and labeling/attribution of musculoskeletal symptoms (e.g., symptoms may be more readily detected in boring, repetitive, narrow jobs where there is little stimulation to compete with symptoms for attention).

Individual factors such as age or gender may modify the effects of physical or work organization/psychosocial demands (e.g., older workers may be more susceptible to injury under conditions of high work demands). Finally, the model recognizes that musculoskeletal outcomes encompass a range of factors, including symptom reporting, health care utilization, and disability.

The data set in the present study contains measures of physical demands, work organization, psychological strain, labeling/attribution, symptoms, health care utilization, and disability. Figure 2 shows the model and pathways that these variables allow us to test. Although several of the pathways listed above are tested, pathways dependent on measurement of biomechanical strain cannot be tested fully given the lack of that measure in the data set.

THE STUDY POPULATION

The data for this analysis come from the Ergonomics and Your Health Project,[19] in which 1779 workers at a large aerospace manufacturing company in the Northeast completed a self-administered survey, on company time, in 1992. The overall response rate was 64%, and data from the questionnaire have been linked with administrative data including workers' compensation and sick hours.

The sample for this analysis excluded nonsalaried or factory/shop floor workers and workers not using a video display terminal (VDT). The response rate for salaried (office) workers, the focus of this analysis, was 65%. A total of 282 women and 523 men completed the questionnaire. A group of 117 salaried engineers were excluded from the analysis because of the inability to reliably define their physical demands. These engineers spent all or none of their time at the VDT depending on whether they were designing a new work process, implementing a new work process, modifying an existing production set-up, or solving a problem on the shop floor. The engineers exclusively worked on the floor or in the office. Excluding this group did not change results and yielded an analytic sample of 249 women and 439 men.

MEASURES USED IN PATH MODELS

This section discusses the specific domains of the ecological model that are depicted in Figure 2.

Physical demands are measured as the amount of time spent during an average week working in front of the VDT. Observers—industrial engineers and occupational safety and health staff—working in the business units where computers were being used determined the amount of time. Individuals were classified into one of five groups (0–29 hours per week, 30–49 hours, 50–79 hours, 80–100 hours, and variable hours). The "variable group" comprised the engineers and was deleted.

Work organization is measured with a set of psychosocial measures.

1. *Job decision latitude* is an index specified by Karasek and is a combination of decision authority (have freedom to make decisions, can choose how to perform work, have a lot of say on the job) and skills discretion (keep learning new things, can develop skills, job requires skill, task variety, repetitious, job requires creativity).[17] It assesses the amount of control a person has over what is done and how it is done.

2. *Psychological job demands* is a measure of the amount of effort required to carry out the work (excessive work, conflicting demands, insufficient time to do work, work fast, work hard) developed by Karasek.[17]

3. *Role ambiguity* is a measure of the lack of clarity in work responsibilities and duties (clear on responsibilities, what others expect of you is predictable, work objectives well defined, clear what others expect) developed by Kahn and colleagues.[9]

4. *Role conflict* is a measure of conflicting demands placed on the worker (people equal in rank and authority, people in a good position to see what you do, and people whose request should be met ask you to do things that conflict) developed by Kahn.[9]

5. *Work-related social support* measures the amount of instrumental and emotional support provided by coworkers and supervisors during the workday (people go out of their way to make work life easier, easy to talk with people, people can be relied upon when things get tough, people willing to listen to personal problems) developed by House.[14,15]

We attempted to reduce the number of work organization measures by examining the intercorrelation between the scales. This led to combining skill discretion and decision authority ($r = 0.65$) into job decision latitude and coworker and supervisor support ($r = 0.40$) into work support based on conceptual congruence. Although psychological job demands and role ambiguities are statistically correlated ($r = 0.42$), we felt they were conceptually different enough to warrant not combining them. The remainder of the correlations were low, ranging from 0.05–0.2.

Psychological strain is measured with two scales. *Global demoralization* is a 27-item nonspecific psychological distress measure developed by Dohrenwend for use in community studies.[11] *Job satisfaction* measures the satisfaction the worker has with 10 facets of the job (job as whole, pay, people work with, boss/supervisor, type of work, chances of promotion, skills use, workstation, tools use, and job security). It is based on earlier Quality of Employment Survey measures.[9]

Individual factors are measured with two variables. *Age* is a continuous measure. *Neuroticism* measures the tendency of a person to report symptoms or other problems in life. It is a 48-item measure developed by Costa and McCrae.[10]

Labeling/Attribution is assessed with a measure of *social desirability*. The 13-item measure is derived from the original 64-item Crowne-Marlowe measure.[29] People who score higher on social desirability tend to try to present themselves in a positive light and are less likely to report symptoms.

Musculoskeletal outcomes are measured in three separate domains.

1. *A symptom/duration measure* was created for each of six musculoskeletal areas (neck, shoulder, elbow, hand/wrist, back, and leg) by multiplying symptom frequency by duration. Each series of questions for a musculoskeletal region has an initial skip question ascertaining the presence or absence of symptoms. Workers reporting no symptoms were assigned a score of zero to retain them in the analysis.

2. *Health care utilization* was measured by combining responses to a series of questions about health care visits (seeing a physician, nurse, physician assistant, nurse practitioner, chiropractor, physical therapist, therapeutic masseuse, surgeon) and treatment (having surgery for current musculoskeletal problem). Weighting facilitated combining the items into a single meaningful scale. Seeing a provider once during the past year was considered much less significant than two to five times (weighted 3) or more than five times (weighted 6). Having surgery was also weighted as 6, and seeing a surgeon was weighted as 3.

3. *Disability* was measured by the number of sick hours in the year following survey administration. The data were obtained through administrative records and are the actual recorded sick hours linked to each individual observation.

TESTING HYPOTHESES USING PATH ANALYSIS

Path analysis forces the person to think ecologically about the effects of office technology on musculoskeletal outcomes. We propose to test the series of hypotheses listed in Table 1; these hypotheses represent the arrows shown in the analytic framework in Figure 2. We leave untested certain hypotheses (e.g., work organization has a direct effect on musculoskeletal symptoms) because we did not feel a priori justification existed; no plausible mechanisms are extant to justify a direct path. All analyses were completed using Stata software.[36] Because preliminary

TABLE 1. Statement of Hypotheses

1. Work organization (lower job decision latitude, lower work support, higher psychological job demands, higher role ambiguity and conflict) is associated with greater levels of video display terminal (VDT) use as a percent of total work time.
2. Work organization, greater VDT use as a percent of total work time, and more neuroticism are associated with higher levels of global demoralization.
3. Work organization, greater VDT use as a percent of total work time, and more neuroticism are associated with lower levels of job satisfaction.
4. Greater VDT use is associated with more social desirability.
5. Greater VDT use, more psychological strain (higher global demoralization, low job satisfaction), more social desirability, and neuroticism are associated with higher levels of musculoskeletal symptom/duration scores.
6. Greater VDT use as a percent of total work time, psychological strain, neuroticism, and higher levels of musculoskeletal symptom/duration scores are associated with more health care utilization due to musculoskeletal problems.
7. Neuroticism, a higher level of musculoskeletal symptom/duration scores, and more health care utilization due to musculoskeletal problems are associated with more sick days.

TABLE 2. Description of Sample: Means for All Variables in Path Models by Gender

	Male (n = 439)	Female (n = 249)
Age	39.4 (9.90)	37.9 (11.20)
Physical demands		
% VDT Use (≥ 50%)	48.7 (50.04)	70.7 (45.61)
Work organization		
Job decision latitude	3.73 (0.64)	3.46 (0.66)
Psychological job demands	3.39 (0.73)	3.39 (0.73)
Role ambiguity	2.09 (0.66)	2.02 (0.68)
Role conflict	1.78 (0.62)	1.77 (0.65)
Work support	15.46 (2.27)	15.63 (2.50)
Individual factor		
Neuroticism	2.34 (0.47)	2.55 (0.51)
Psychological strain		
Global demoralization	0.75 (0.45)	0.95 (0.56)
Job satisfaction	2.88 (0.49)	2.90 (0.51)
Social desirability		
Social desirability	1.68 (0.20)	1.70 (0.21)
Musculoskeletal symptom/duration		
Neck region	3.74 (6.21)	7.33 (3.75)
Shoulder region	2.60 (5.83)	4.79 (9.21)
Elbow region	1.56 (4.67)	2.10 (5.90)
Hand region	2.51 (5.54)	5.43 (8.18)
Back region	4.38 (6.56)	6.99 (9.15)
Leg region	3.70 (7.41)	4.44 (8.01)
Health care utilization associated with		
Neck problems	1.12 (2.94)	1.95 (4.71)
Shoulder problems	1.53 (3.00)	2.64 (4.72)
Elbow problems	0.90 (2.03)	1.80 (3.35)
Hand problems	1.09 (2.88)	2.09 (4.04)
Back problems	1.66 (3.14)	2.12 (3.88)
Leg problems	2.08 (3.95)	2.71 (4.60)
Disability		
Sick hours	11.92 (24.07)	25.72 (42.72)

( ) = Standard deviation, VDT = video display terminal

analyses revealed gender differences in findings, all results are presented by gender. Table 2 shows all variables used in the path analysis by gender.

To test the ecological framework, we used path analysis by multiple linear regression.[3] Testing for the significance of any path is a parsimonious way of hypothesis testing.[2] A significance level of 0.05 was considered appropriate for this preliminary test. Indirect and direct effects are calculated providing estimates of the total effect (the sum of the direct and indirect—the product of all effects along a path—effects) for each office and individual domain to the musculoskeletal outcomes.[27] The utility of path analysis resides not only in its ability to partition variance but in testing the appropriateness of the structure of the model.[12]

We present our findings as a series of path diagrams for men and women with the significant direct effects shown. All the variables are standardized (subtract mean and divide by standard deviation) before being entered into the regression equations. Six separate regression models were estimated for men and women. Because of the high intercorrelation between demoralization and neuroticism (r = 0.74), entering both in one model causes collinearity problems. Thus, neuroticism is only included in models with job satisfaction. Because multiple measures of work organization and psychological strain are used, we present multiple findings within single-path diagrams. Age was considered the only significant confounder and therefore is introduced in all models. There are few differences between models. Where differences exist (e.g., two significant correlations differing by 0.03), we report the lower value. Thus, our effect estimates are conservative.

FINDINGS

Paths to Individual Psychological States

Work organization does not predict physical demands for men or women (Fig. 3). Physical demands do not predict global demoralization or job satisfaction. Psychosocial work organization predicts global demoralization and job satisfaction. For each measure the relationship is as predicted; for example, positive aspects of work organization are positively associated with job satisfaction and negatively associated with demoralization. Two measures used in job strain research—job decision latitude and psychological

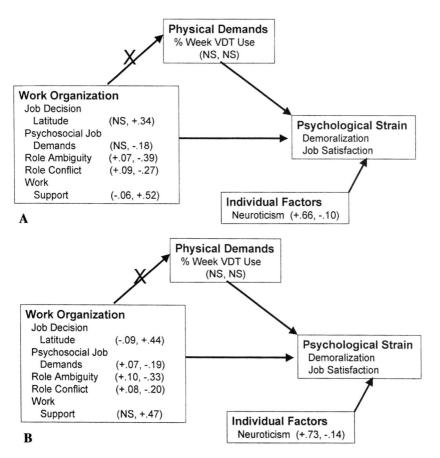

FIGURE 3. Paths from office technology to psychological strain outcomes. **A,** For men (n = 439). **B,** For women (n = 249). Path coefficients for demoralization and satisfaction are in parentheses. X = no significant effects for specified path, VDT = video display terminal, NS = not significant.

job demands—did not predict demoralization for men.[18] Neuroticism was very highly correlated with global demoralization (partial correlation ranges 0.6–0.7).

Paths to Musculoskeletal Outcomes

Musculoskeletal symptom/duration outcomes are not predicted by percent VDT use or social desirability for men or women (Fig. 4). The lack of a relationship between physical demands and VDT use is counterintuitive, because research has shown using the VDT for at least half of the day predicts musculoskeletal disorders (WRMDs). In fact, in other analyses of this data set where a more restrictive case definition for WRMDs was used, greater than 50% VDT use increased the risk of hand/wrist WRMDs by 87%.[19] In our analysis we did not adopt the National Institute for Occupational Safety and Health's criteria for defining a self-reported case of WRMDs, e.g., excluding workers who report that the symptoms were not work-related and did not occur on the current job.[23] This has

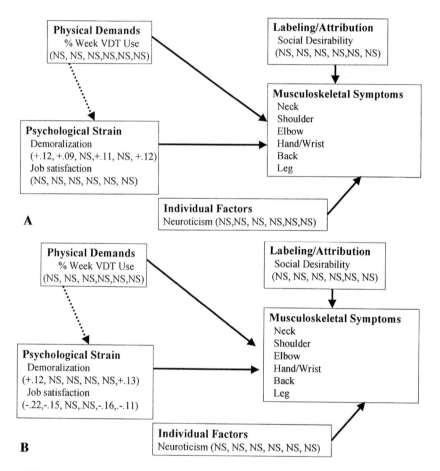

FIGURE 4. Paths from physical demands and psychological strains to musculoskeletal symptom/duration outcomes. **A,** For men (n = 439). **B,** For women (n = 249). The path coefficients (in parentheses) from left to right are for each musculoskeletal region from neck to leg. Dashed arrow = a path whose effects have been shown in a prior figure, VDT = video display terminal, NS = not significant.

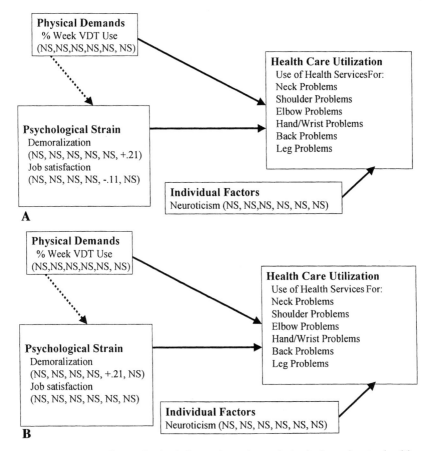

FIGURE 5.   Paths from physical demands and psychological strains to health care utilization outcomes due to musculoskeletal injuries. **A**, For men (n = 439). **B**, For women (n = 249). The path coefficients (in parentheses) from left to right are for each musculoskeletal region from neck to leg. Dashed arrow = a path whose effects have been shown in a prior figure, VDT = video display terminal, NS = not significant.

the potential to attenuate the effects of work. In future analyses we intend to separate the effects of nonwork demands through the introduction of new paths.

Global demoralization predicts neck and leg symptoms for both men and women; the higher the general psychiatric morbidity, the higher the level of symptom/duration. Men who are demoralized are more likely to report shoulder and hand/wrist symptoms. Job dissatisfaction is a strong predictor of neck, shoulder, back, and leg symptoms for women but not men.

Health care utilization associated with musculoskeletal injuries is not predicted by physical demands, psychological strain, or neuroticism for men or women (Fig. 5) For men demoralization predicts health care use associated with leg symptoms, while job dissatisfaction predicts back symptom health care utilization. Musculoskeletal symptoms predict health care utilization for both men and women (Fig. 6). Women with hand/wrist symptoms are more likely to seek health care, but there is no significant relationship for men ($\beta = 0.061$, $p = 0.253$).

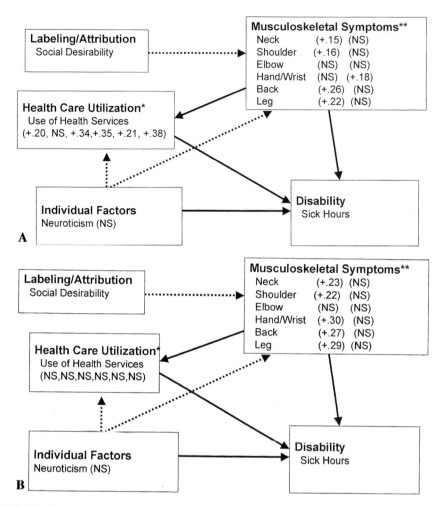

FIGURE 6. Paths from musculoskeletal symptom/duration and health care utilization to disability. **A**, For men (n = 439). **B**, For women (n = 249). * The path coefficients correspond to the unique effect of each musculoskeletal region on sick hours. ** The first column of path coefficients corresponds to the impact of each symptom on health care use; the second of each symptom on sick hours. Dashed arrow = a path whose effects have been shown in a prior figure, NS = not significant.

Disability, measured by sick hours, is predicted by health care utilization **only** for men. Health care use associated with all musculoskeletal regions except the shoulder is associated with more sick hours. Musculoskeletal symptoms do not directly predict sick hours for men or women; rather, they indirectly influence sick hours for men through health care use.

Estimating the Total Impact on Musculoskeletal Outcomes

An advantage to path analysis is that you can estimate direct and indirect effects. In this chapter we are interested in the direct and indirect effects of work organization

TABLE 3.   Summary of Direct and Indirect Effects in Path Models for Hand/Wrist Musculoskeletal Region for Men and Women

	Men								
	Effects on Symptoms			Effects on Health Care Use			Effects on Disability		
	Direct	Indirect	Total	Direct	Indirect	Total	Direct	Indirect	Total
VDT use	0.0322	0.0028	0.0349	0.0320	0.0026	0.0346		0.0180	0.0180
Role ambiguity		0.0117	0.0117		0.0045	0.0045		0.0036	0.0036
Neuroticism		0.0761	0.0761		0.0103	0.0103	0.0076	0.0168	0.0245
Global demoralization	0.1140		0.1140	0.0077	0.0077	0.0154		0.0252	0.0252
Social desirability	-0.0100		-0.0100		-0.0007	-0.0007		-0.0020	-0.0020
Musculoskeletal symptoms				0.0677		0.0677	0.1747	0.0234	0.1981
Health care use								0.3448	0.3448

	Women								
	Effects on Symptoms			Effects on Health Care Use			Effects on Disability		
	Direct	Indirect	Total	Direct	Indirect	Total	Direct	Indirect	Total
VDT use	0.0867	-0.0047	0.0820	0.0413	0.0246	0.0659		0.0132	0.0132
Role ambiguity		0.0056	0.0056		0.0011	0.0011		0.0008	0.0008
Neuroticism		0.0616	0.0616		0.0229	0.0229	0.2275	0.0089	0.2365
Global demoralization	0.0834		0.0834	0.0057	0.0253	0.0310		0.0121	0.0121
Social desirability	-0.0150		-0.0150		-0.0046	-0.0046		-0.0021	-0.0021
Musculoskeletal symptoms				0.3037		0.3037	0.1312	0.0115	0.1426
Health care use							0.0378		0.0378

Note: Total effects are the sum of the direct and indirect effects.
VDT = video display terminal

and physical demands on musculoskeletal symptoms, health care use associated with musculoskeletal symptoms, and sick hours. We do not present all effects but have chosen several illustrative paths. We choose only two musculoskeletal regions (hand/wrist and back), one work organization factor (role ambiguity), and one psychological strain (global demoralization) to illustrate the total effects. Care should be taken in interpreting effect sizes in Tables 3 and 4 because paths contributing to an effect may be nonsignificant even though correlations are large. Below, we point out instances where this occurs.

MUSCULOSKELETAL SYMPTOMS

For men global demoralization has the largest total effect on hand/wrist symptom/duration scores (Table 3). While VDT use and global demoralization have similar effects on musculoskeletal symptoms among women, the paths used to calculate effects are nonsignificant (see Figs. 3 and 4). A similar pattern of effects exists for the back musculoskeletal region (Table 4).

HEALTH CARE USE

For women health care use associated with hand/wrist problems is being driven by hand/wrist musculoskeletal symptom/duration scores (see Table 3). The effect of VDT use among women is comparable to the effect of musculoskeletal symptom/duration scores for men, illustrating a striking gender difference; again, these paths are nonsignificant. All other effects are small. For both men and women with

TABLE 4.   Summary of Direct and Indirect Effects in Path Models for Back Musculoskeletal Region for Men and Women

	Men								
	Effects on Symptoms			Effects on Health Care Use			Effects on Disability		
	Direct	Indirect	Total	Direct	Indirect	Total	Direct	Indirect	Total
VDT use	0.0255	0.0017	0.0272	-0.0159	0.0089	-0.0070		0.0015	0.0015
Role ambiguity		0.0078	0.0078		0.0057	0.0057		0.0021	0.0021
Neuroticism							0.0080	-0.0216	-0.0296
Global demoralization	0.0715		0.0715	0.0684	0.0192	0.0876		0.0266	0.0266
Social desirability	0.0037		0.0037		0.0010	0.0010		0.0006	0.0006
Musculoskeletal symptoms				0.2682		0.2682	0.1103	0.0575	0.1678
Health care use							0.2143		0.2143
	Women								
	Effects on Symptoms			Effects on Health Care Use			Effects on Disability		
	Direct	Indirect	Total	Direct	Indirect	Total	Direct	Indirect	Total
VDT use	-0.1028	-0.0055	-0.1083	0.0194	-0.0406	-0.0212		0.0005	0.0005
Role ambiguity		0.0124	0.0124		0.0231	0.0231		-0.0009	-0.0009
Neuroticism		0.0725	0.0725		0.1741	0.1714	0.1353	-0.0069	0.1284
Global demoralization	0.0981		0.0981	0.2096	0.0261	0.2357		-0.0093	-0.0093
Social desirability	0.0042		0.0042		0.0011	0.0011		0.0000	0.0000
Musculoskeletal symptoms				0.2658		0.2658	0.0030	-0.0108	-0.0079
Health care use							-0.0407		-0.0407

Note: Total effects are the sum of the direct and indirect effects.
VDT = video display terminal

back problems, musculoskeletal symptom/duration scores drive health care use (see Table 4). However, for women with back problems demoralization is a major effect along with the symptom/duration scores. While the effect size for neuroticism among women is large, we emphasize the nonsignificance of this factor in the path models.

DISABILITY

For men health care use associated with hand/wrist problems is driving sick hours (see Table 3). For women the major effect is with hand/wrist musculoskeletal symptoms/duration scores. For back musculoskeletal problems, sick hours or lost productivity is driven by both health care use associated with back problems and the back symptom/duration scores in men (see Table 4).

DISCUSSION AND IMPLICATIONS

We proposed and tested an ecological model for understanding the origins of musculoskeletal injuries.[32] Work organization has consistent effects on psychological strain but small total effects on musculoskeletal symptoms, health care utilization, and disability for men and on musculoskeletal symptoms and health care use for women. The patterns of effects do not vary substantially across musculoskeletal regions for office workers, potentially indicating a general influence of work organization, i.e., work organization would not be expected to target a specific body region. This is consistent with findings of other studies.[5,13,20]

A well-validated measure of social desirability did not relate to the symptom/duration measure. This finding was consistent across musculoskeletal regions. A striking finding is the **lack** of strong and consistent neuroticism effects. McCrae and Costa describe neuroticism as a stable trait of adult life that reflects a person's tendency to report certain types of symptoms.[22] Although strongly related to global demoralization for both men and women, neuroticism was only modestly associated with musculoskeletal symptoms. The lack of a gender difference builds on earlier work to suggest that worker reports of musculoskeletal symptoms and health care use are not influenced by this underlying personality trait.[19]

The path models show that health care use associated with musculoskeletal injuries is not determined by mental health or individual traits that may lead one to seek care. Rather, symptoms drive health care utilization; the higher the level of symptom/duration, the more likely the worker will seek care. The implication for employers and practitioners is that to reduce health care costs they must reduce musculoskeletal injuries through job redesign, ergonomics, or changes in work scheduling.

The gender difference in the relationship between lost productivity as measured by sick hours was surprising. While WRMDs, especially of the hand/wrist, are more prevalent among women, this does not translate into greater lost productivity. These findings are strengthened by the prospective relationship between symptoms and lost productivity. While we have no data to account for the lack of relationship between health care use and sick hours for women, there are several plausible reasons for the observed effect:

- Use of onsite health services that do not require use of sick time could be higher among women.
- Because women seek treatment for symptoms earlier than men, their treatment for symptoms may not require extended absences.[37]
- Women, in general, are more likely to use sick time for family care, which could explain why women have a higher mean sick hour usage (see Table 2) not related to health care use associated with musculoskeletal symptoms.[6]

There are several limitations to the current analysis. For example, the cross-sectional design precludes the examining of temporal ordering (e.g., to definitively state psychological strain is producing musculoskeletal symptoms rather than the reverse). Additionally, physical demands are measured in a limited way, and biomechanical strain measures are absent.

Implications for Research

Musculoskeletal cumulative trauma disorders are difficult to diagnose, and there is continued debate on the most appropriate case definition. Musculoskeletal injuries as a class of injuries have many causes. These factors make the conduct of epidemiologic studies more challenging.[19] Future research should (1) incorporate a double-blind prospective design in which subjects are recruited prior to exposure and disease; (2) attempt to develop new measures of work organization that capture the important elements of computer-mediated work (e.g., cognitive demands, online communication and support); (3) develop more complete assessments of the range of musculoskeletal outcomes (e.g., using workers' compensation and functional health measures of disability); and (4) incorporate nonwork demands into the model.

The use of multiple indicators of musculoskeletal outcomes is a new approach to understanding the broader health impact of office environments. Perhaps the single most important new development is the multiple pathways uncovered between musculoskeletal symptom/duration, health care use, and sick days. This linkage has direct implications for the cost of doing business and should be a central research topic in the future. While there may never be resolution on the measurement of WRMD cases, showing the cost drivers and nondrivers will help in business decisions.

Implications for Intervention

The data do not strongly support reducing the amount of time at VDTs as a method for reducing musculoskeletal outcomes or lost productivity due to disability. While there is a dose-response relationship between VDT use and musculoskeletal symptoms,[28] recent research indicates that this relationship can be modified by work organization interventions such as more frequent rest breaks.[34]

Clearly the broader ecological model identifies the importance of preventing injuries to reduce health care costs and lost productivity. This is supported by our findings that symptoms—not VDT use, neuroticism, or psychological strain—are linked with health care utilization and lost productivity. Therefore, interventions targeting reduction of symptom development are needed. Although the role of psychological strain in musculoskeletal symptom/duration experience is well described,[4,5,13,33] the key predictors of psychological strain in our model are not easily changed without more widespread organizational change.

The role of providers in health care delivery can be important, as the gender differences shown in Figure 6 illustrate. Why men and women show these differences in lost productivity are intriguing. While there is much literature on differential treatment of men and women by providers, this probably does not explain the observed gender differences. Rather, women may choose to use sick hours to manage family crises rather than for injuries that did not require immediate attention. This suggests that the appropriate interventions are changes to the benefits programs to provide other supports for family crises. Given the known gender differences in health care behavior, encouraging all workers with symptoms to seek care earlier rather than changing provider behavior could be critical in reducing the impact of symptoms on lost productivity. An alternative may be to train supervisors and give them incentives to encourage workers to seek care when symptoms begin instead of waiting until they can no longer work.

ACKNOWLEDGEMENT

The authors wish to thank the Office Ergonomics Research Committee, the National Institute for Occupational Safety and Health, and the National Institute for Aging for support in preparing this chapter.

REFERENCES

1. Amick BC III, Celentano DD: Human factors epidemiology: An integrated approach for the study of health issues. In Cohen BGF (ed): Office Work in Human Aspects of Office Automation. Amsterdam, Elsevier Press, 1984, pp 362–394.
2. Amick BC III, Celentano DD: Structural determinants of the psychosocial work environment: Introducing technology in the work stress framework. Ergonomics 34:625–646, 1991.
3. Asher HB: Causal Modeling. Beverly Hills, CA, Sage Publications, 1976.
4. Bergqvist U, Wolgast E, Nilsson B, Voss M: Musculoskeletal disorders among visual display terminal workers: Individual ergonomic and work organizational factors. Ergonomics 38:763–776, 1995.
5. Bernard B, Sauter SL, Fine LJ, et al: Psychosocial and work organization risk factors for cumulative trauma disorders in the hands and wrists of newspaper employees. Scand J Work Environ Health 18(suppl 2):119–120, 1992.
6. Bond JT, Galinsky E, Swanburg JE: The 1997 National Study of the Changing Workforce. New York, Families and Work Institute, 1997.

7. Bongers PM, De Winter CR, Kompier MJ, Hildebrandt VH: Psychosocial factors and work and musculoskeletal disease. Scand J Work Environ Health 19:297–312, 1993.
8. Cakir A, Hart DJ, Stewart DFM: Research into the Effects of Video Display Workplaces on the Physical and Psychological Function of Persons. Bonn, West Germany, Federal Ministry for Work and Social Order, 1978.
9. Caplan R, Cobb S, French JR, et al: Job Demands and Worker Health. Washington, DC, National Institute for Occupational Safety and Health, 1975, 75-160.
10. Costa P, McCrae R: NEO PI-R Professional Manual. Odessa, FL, PAR Press, 1992.
11. Dohrenwend BP, Levav I, Shrout PE: Screening scales for the psychiatric epidemiology research interview (PERI). In Weissman MM, Myers JK, Ross CE (eds): Community Surveys of Psychiatric Disorders. New Brunswick, NJ, Rutgers University Press, 1986, pp 349–375.
12. Duncan OD: Partials, partitions and paths. In Borgatta EF, Bohrnstedt GW (eds): Sociological Methodology. San Francisco, Jossey-Bass, 1970, pp 79–109.
13. Hoekstra E, Hurrell J, Swanson N: Evaluation of work-related musculoskeletal disorders and job stress among teleservice center representatives. Appl Occup Environ Hyg 10:812–817, 1995.
14. House J: Work Stress and Social Support. Reading, MA, Addison-Wesley, 1981.
15. House J: The America's Changing Lives Survey. Ann Arbor, MI, Institute for Survey Research, University of Michigan, 1992.
16. Hunting W, Laubli T, Grandjean E: Postural and visual loads at VDT workplaces. I. Constrained postures. Ergonomics 24:917–931, 1981.
17. Karasek R: The Job Content Questionnaire User's Guide. Lowell, MA, Department of Work Environment, University of Massachusetts, 1991.
18. Karasek RA, Theorell T: Healthy Work: Stress Productivity and the Reconstruction of Working Life. New York, Basic Books, 1990.
19. Kasl SV, Amick BC III: Cumulative trauma disorder research: Methodological issues and illustrative findings from the perspective of psychosocial epidemiology. In Moon S, Sauter S (eds): Psychosocial Factors and Musculoskeletal Disorders in Office Work. New York, Taylor and Francis, 1996, pp 263–284.
20. Linton SJ, Kamwendo K: Risk factors in the psychosocial work environment for neck and shoulder pain in secretaries. J Occup Med 31:609–613, 1989.
21. Maeda K, Hunting W, Grandjean E: Localized fatigue in accounting-machine operators. J Occup Med 22:810–816, 1980.
22. McCrae RR, Costa PT Jr: Personality in Adulthood. New York, The Guilford Press, 1990.
23. National Institute for Occupational Safety and Health: US West Communications Health Hazard Evaluation Report. Cincinnati, NIOSH, 1992, HETA 89-299-2230.
24. National Institute for Occupational Safety and Health: National Occupational Research Agenda. Cincinnati, NIOSH, 1996, publication 96-115.
25. Ong CN, Hoong BT, Phoon WO: Visual and muscular fatigue in operators using visual display terminals. J Hum Ergol (Tokyo) 10:161–171, 1981.
26. Onishi N, Normura H, Sakai K: Fatigue and strength of upper limb muscles of flight reservation system operators. J Hum Ergol (Tokyo) 2:133–141, 1973.
27. Pedhazur EJ: Multiple Regression in Behavioral Research. New York, CBS College Publishing, 1982.
28. Punnett L, Bergqvist U: Video display unit work and upper extremity musculoskeletal disorders: A review of epidemiologic findings. In Work and Health Scientific Series, 16. Solna, Sweden, National Institute for Working Life, 1997, pp 1–161.
29. Reynolds W: Development of reliable and valid short forms of the Marlowe-Crowne social desirability scale. J Clin Psychol 38:119–125, 1982.
30. Sauter SL, Schleifer LM, Knutson SJ: Work posture workstation design and musculoskeletal discomfort in a VDT data entry task. Hum Factors 33:151–167, 1991.
31. Sauter SL: Ergonomics stress and the redesign of office work. Presented at the National Occupational Musculoskeletal Injury Conference, Ann Arbor, MI, April 1991.
32. Sauter SL, Swanson NG: An ecological model of musculoskeletal disorders in office work. In Moon S, Sauter SL (eds): Beyond Biomechanics: Psychosocial Aspects of Musculoskeletal Disorders in Office Work. London, Taylor & Francis, 1996, pp 3–21.
33. Sauter SL, Gottlieb MS, Jones KC, et al: Job and health implications of VDT use: Initial results of the Wisconsin-NIOSH study. Communications of the Association for Computing Machinery 26:284–294, 1983.
34. Sauter S, Swanson N, Conway F, et al: Prospective study of rest break interventions in keyboard intensive work. Proceedings of the Marconi Research Conference, Marshall, CA, April 13–16, 1997.

35. Smith MJ, Carayon P: Work organization stress and cumulative trauma disorders. In Moon SD, Sauter SL (eds): Beyond Biomechanics: Psychosocial Aspects of Musculoskeletal Disorders in Office Work. London, Taylor & Francis, 1996, pp 23–42.

36. StataCorp: Stata Statistical Software: Release 5.0. College Station, TX, Stata Corporation, 1997.

37. Walsh DC, Sorensen G, Leonard L: Gender, health, and cigarette smoking. In Amick BC, Levine S, Tarlov AR, Walsh DC (eds): Society & Health. New York, Oxford University Press, 1995, pp 131–171.

LAURA PUNNETT, ScD
ULF BERGQVIST, DrMedSci, MSci Tech

MUSCULOSKELETAL DISORDERS IN VISUAL DISPLAY UNIT WORK: GENDER AND WORK DEMANDS

From the Department of Work
Environment
University of Massachusetts
Lowell, Massachusetts
and
National Institute of Working Life
Solna, Sweden

Reprint requests to:
Laura Punnett, ScD
Department of Work Environment
One University Avenue
University of Massachusetts Lowell
Lowell, MA 01854

Concerns about adverse health problems among users of visual display units (VDUs) have been voiced since they came into widespread use in the mid 1970s. Ergonomic factors have been a central issue from the beginning, in part due to accumulating knowledge about their health hazards in general.[1] Relevant features of the work environment related to the new technology included equipment, workstation dimensions, increasingly stereotyped and repetitive manual motion patterns, increased monotony, and decreased decision latitude in the job. The risk of upper extremity musculoskeletal disorders (MSDs) continues to be a primary concern among VDU users, and the relationship of these disorders with VDU work now has been relatively well documented.[2]

Being female is often described as a risk factor for MSDs, but this observation is not specific to VDU work. In addition to the physical differences between men and women, gender is a social construct. Gender differences in health may be confounded by occupational demands, such as more immobility at workstations and more repetitive motion patterns,[3] more monotonous work content, or lower job decision latitude:[4] such differences in exposure may be found even within job titles.[5] Gender also may serve as a proxy for differences between men and women in the amount and type of household work, levels of psychosocial strain outside the work environment, or types of recreational activities.

However, despite sex segregation in workplaces worldwide, there have been a few opportunities to compare the frequency of MSDs among women and men with similar work demands. For example, after controlling for job demands, Silverstein et al. found that women had an increased risk of hand/wrist disorders compared to men; most of the gender difference appeared to occur in jobs with high manual forces but low repetitiveness, a situation in which few female subjects were employed.[6] However, for the more specific outcome of carpal tunnel syndrome, there was no effect of gender once the effect of physical job demands was taken into account.[7] Other researchers also have shown that men and women have similar health effects when employed in similar working conditions.[8,9] Thus, the epidemiologic associations of MSDs with occupational ergonomic exposures must be analyzed separately by gender to determine whether women are at higher risk than men when exposed to the same or similar levels of occupational ergonomic stressors.

The possible differences between men and women in the risk of upper extremity and neck MSDs related to VDU work can be described in two different but complementary ways:

- Do women working with VDUs have a higher occurrence of such disorders than men who work with VDUs? In other words, is gender—or factors related to gender—a risk factor for such disorders, conditional on or adjusting for ergonomic exposures?
- Is the risk associated with VDU work different for men and women, i.e., is gender an effect modifier for occupational exposures, whether biomechanical or psychosocial?

To the extent that there is a gender differential in the frequency of occurrence or the risk of MSDs, how should it be interpreted? Gender involves biologic differences, at least on average, in parameters as diverse as strength capacity and endocrine hormone levels. As a social construct, gender presents many implications for life at work and outside of work. Thus, in addition to physiologic differences between men and women, many of which are of unknown relevance to the cause of MSDs, there are likely differences in pain reporting and medical care-seeking behavior, in job assignments and consequent ergonomic exposures in paid work and work in the home, and in strategies for performing different types of physical work. Using gender as a variable to evaluate or adjust for the difference between men and women in a study does not, by itself, help to clarify these possible explanations.

ERGONOMIC EXPOSURES AND RISK OF UPPER EXTREMITY MUSCULOSKELETAL DISORDERS

Work at a VDU may involve several physical actions that have been cited as risk factors for MSDs, including stereotyped repetition of manual motion patterns, rapid work pace, dynamic and static anatomically nonneutral body postures, and mechanical stress concentrations, or direct pressure of hard surfaces or sharp edges on soft body tissues. There is substantial epidemiologic, physiologic, and biomechanical evidence showing the effects of these stressors on the soft tissues of the musculoskeletal system[1] (see David Rempel's chapter).

Different types of VDU work present different kinds of physical and mental demands, such as the amount of data input performed or amount of visual information processing. The categories proposed originally by the National Research Council have often been used as an appropriate characterization of different task designs: "data entry," "data acquisition," "interactive communication," "word processing," and "programming, computer-assisted design (CAD), and computer assisted manufacturing."[10]

These categories represent differences in objectives, work content and autonomy, and physical features of the job, such as speed of keying, lack of variability in motion patterns, and frequency and duration of rest breaks.

Another type of stressor that has received increasing interest with respect to MSDs is psychosocial factors in the workplace. The psychological and social dimensions of the work environment are commonly divided into the following categories, mainly based on work by Karasek and colleagues:[4]

- The psychological demands of the job, including the amount of work and the time available to complete it
- The worker's opportunities to exercise control in the job, often defined as job control or decision latitude
- The degree of social support by supervisors and coworkers
- Job insecurity, the worker's fear of being replaced, or perceived opportunities for future employment and advancement

These psychosocial factors often occur as consequences of objectively definable work organization features such as task allocation and specialization, incentive wages, and work pace. They have been demonstrated epidemiologically to have etiologic importance for cardiovascular disease.[4] Their role in the development of MSDs is plausible on the basis of known physiologic mechanisms, such as adverse circulatory patterns, sympathetic nervous symptom arousal, tonic activation or psychogenic muscular tension, and interference with normal muscle and tendon repair processes. The epidemiologic literature on this question is evolving; to date, decision latitude, or autonomy, is the psychosocial stressor most consistently associated with MSDs.[11]

However, the extent to which occupational psychosocial factors are independent risk factors for MSDs or primarily have an effect in the presence of physical exposures remains to be clarified.[12] The common distinction between physical and psychosocial ergonomic risk factors is troubling in light of the substantial overlap between many of these features as experienced by workers. For example, high psychological work demands typically require rapid physical work pace and cause the operator to feel pressured; highly stereotyped finger motion patterns occur when the job is monotonous and offers little decision autonomy.

In a recent review of the epidemiology of upper extremity MSDs in VDU users, we evaluated the published literature according to standard epidemiologic criteria.[2] Of 51 etiologic studies on this topic, 25 met the specified methodologic criteria and could be relied upon to draw conclusions. All 25 studies either used statistical techniques to adjust for the effect of gender or restricted the study population to women. There was strong evidence for a dose-response relationship between risk of hand and wrist disorders and hours of keying per day.[13,14] MSD occurrence was influenced by organizational aspects of modern office work, such as data entry and other intensive keying tasks and the increased speed of handling calls by telephone operators.[15] The literature also showed an elevated risk of upper extremity disorders among VDU users with poor workstation layout and resulting postural strain. Eight of nine intervention studies showed at least some reduction in frequency of MSD symptoms, examination findings, or absenteeism after implementation of workplace ergonomic interventions, including workstation and chair redesign and the training of workers.

Of the literature that addressed psychosocial features of VDU jobs, a few studies demonstrated associations between MSDs and decision latitude, social support, and job insecurity or job dissatisfaction; one reported interactions between psychosocial factors and poor workstation features. However, the overall evidence was inconsistent and presented several difficulties in interpretation of the results, in particular because so many of the studies reviewed were cross-sectional and thus could not determine whether psychosocial stressors had preceded MSD onset or whether onset had caused the worker to experience the psychological and social work environment differently.

The level, frequency, and duration of exposure to ergonomic stressors in VDU jobs may vary, both within and among workplaces. Although the extent to which their variability is associated with gender has been poorly studied, some data are available regarding differences in types of VDU tasks often performed by men and women. For example, Evans collected almost 4,000 responses from VDU users to a magazine survey.[16] Although the utility of the data is limited by possible selection bias, there were substantial gender differences in the types of VDU work performed: men performed a greater variety of VDU tasks, used the VDU fewer hours per day, and worked fewer hours continuously without a break.

GENDER DIFFERENCES IN MSD RISK AND IN EXPOSURES

Many of the methodologically stronger studies provided data that could be used to compare the risk of upper extremity MSDs between male and female VDU operators. Three of six investigations showed a substantial excess of neck or shoulder discomforts among women compared to men (Table 1). Gender differences were less notable for the distal extremity; only one study found a higher risk among women for elbow symptoms, and two found higher risk for the wrist/hand (Table 2). The

TABLE 1. Odds Ratios (95% Confidence Intervals) for Musculoskeletal Symptoms of the Upper Torso in Women Compared to Men Employed in Video Display Unit (VDU) Work

Study author, Date	Study Population	Neck Symptoms	Shoulder Symptoms	Recall Period of Symptoms
Aronsson, 1992	General VDU	2.2 (1.8–2.7)	2.8 (2.3–3.6)	Last 12 months (cOR)
	Routine VDU	1.5 (1.0–2.2)	2.2 (1.4–3.4)	Last 12 months (cOR)
	CAD or programming work	2.9 (1.6–5.5)	3.1 (1.6–5.8)	
Bergqvist, Wolgast, Nilsson & Voss, 1995	Routine VDU	1.3 (0.7–2.3)*	1.3 (0.7–2.3)*	Last 12 months (cOR)
Bernard, 1994	General VDU	2.1 (1.4–2.4)	2.2 (1.5–3.3)	Last 12 months (aOR)
	VDU jobs with similar gender distribution	1.9 (0.8–4.5)	1.5 (0.5–4.8)	Last 12 months (aOR)
Burt, 1990	Newspaper workers	2.3 (1.5–3.5)	1.3 (p = 0.15)	Last 12 months (neck: aOR, shoulder: cOR)
Hales, 1992	Various telecommunication workers	No association (p > 0.05)	No association (p > 0.05)	
Polanyi, 1997	Newspaper workers	2.2 (1.5–3.3)**		Last 12 months (aOR): neck, shoulder, elbow, or wrist/hand
SHARP, 1993	Billing clerks (routine work)	OR not given (p > 0.05)	OR not given (p > 0.05)	Last 12 months (aOR)

OR = odds radios comparing women with men; cOR = crude OR (no adjustments for other variables); aOR = adjusted OR for other variables; ND = not determined or reported; CAD = computer assisted design; SHARP = Safety and Health Assessment & Research For Prevention
* Neck and shoulder discomforts reported together   ** All upper extremity regions combined

TABLE 2.   Odds Ratios (95% Confidence Intervals) for Musculoskeletal Symptoms of the Distal Extremity in Women Compared to Men Employed in Video Display Unit (VDU) Work

Study author, Date	Study Population	Elbow Symptoms	Hand/Wrist Symptoms	Recall Period of Symptoms
Aronsson, 1992	General VDU	2.3 (1.5–3.7)	2.5 (1.8–3.6)	Last 12 months (cOR)
Bergqvist, Wolgast, Nilsson & Voss, 1995	Routine VDU	ND	1.1* (0.6–2.2)	Last 12 months (cOR)
Bernard, 1994	General VDU	ND	1.7 (1.2–2.4)	Last 12 months (aOR)
	VDU work with similar gender occupancy	ND	1.7 (0.8–3.6)	Last 12 months (aOR)
Burt, 1990	Newspaper workers	1.3 (p = 0.26)	1.2 (0.9–1.7)	Last 12 months (cOR)
Hales, 1992	Various telecom-munication workers	No association (p > 0.05)	No association (p > 0.05)	
SHARP, 1993	Billing clerks (routine work)	OR not given (p > 0.05)	OR not given (p > 0.05)	Last 12 months (aOR)

OR = odds radios comparing women with men; cOR = crude OR (no adjustments for other variables); aOR = adjusted OR for other variables; ND = not determined or reported; SHARP = Safety and Health Assessment & Research For Prevention
* Arm and hand discomforts reported together

SHARP study[17] showed a higher crude prevalence among women that was not statistically significant, but that may have reflected the fact that the study included only 11 men. In a seventh paper, published after our review, MSDs affecting any part of the upper limb were studied among newspaper employees using VDUs.[18] More symptoms were reported in the neck and shoulder than in the elbow or wrist/hand, and the prevalence in all regions combined was twice as high among women as men (see Table 1).

Bergqvist's study was carried out at workplaces with a high degree of routine work for both men and women,[19] which is somewhat unusual among studies of VDU work. The similar prevalences found in men and women suggest that gender differences observed in other studies may actually represent differences in type of work, which did not exist in this population. Some support for this explanation is found in studies by Aronsson et al. and Bernard et al., where smaller gender differences for neck and shoulder problems were found when the study population was limited to men and women with more routine work or with more comparable jobs.[20,21]

However, in a prior investigation of the same population studied by Bergqvist et al., Knave and coworkers found higher discomfort scores (frequency and intensity) for women compared to men in the neck, shoulder, upper arm, elbow, forearm, and hand.[22] Furthermore, the opposite trend to that of Bergqvist's results was found by Aronsson et al.[20] when examining professional (CAD/programming) work (see Table 1). Although there was no detectable difference between men and women in the prevalence of disorders in the study by Hales et al., female gender had a weak positive association with a neck/shoulder symptom score that combined severity, frequency, and duration.[23,24]

Few studies reported the influence of other factors on these gender-specific odds ratios. For example, in the study by Bernard et al., the odds ratios for neck, shoulder, and hand/wrist symptoms were adjusted for a number of job tasks and psychological and social factors.[21] However, because crude gender odds ratios were not

TABLE 3.   Odds Ratios (95% Confidence Intervals) for Musculoskeletal Diagnoses in Women Compared to Men Employed in Video Display Unit (VDU) Work

Study author, Date	Study Population	Tension Neck Syndrome	Cervical Disorders	Any Shoulder Diagnosis	Any Arm/Hand Diagnosis	Comments
Bergqvist, Wolgast, Nilsson & Voss, 1995	Routine VDU work	2.2 (1.0–4.9)	1.3 (0.6–2.7)	5.1 (1.2–45)	7.4 (1.1–311)	cOR
	Routine VDU work; women with children at home*	6.4 (1.9–22)	ND	7.1 (1.6–32)	5.2 (1.2–2.3)	aOR
Bozi Ferraz, 1995	Routine VDU work	2.6 (1.2–5.9)**				cOR
Hales, 1992, 1994	General VDU work	Neck ($p < 0.05$) and shoulder ($p < 0.05$) associated with gender in crude analysis; gender not associated with any of the four upper extremity disorders in the final model				aOR

OR = odds ratios comparing women with men; cOR = crude OR (no adjustments for other variables); aOR = adjusted OR for other variables; ND = not determined or reported

* For women without children at home, the aOR was not significantly different than for men; e.g., for tension neck syndrome, the aOR was 2.0 (0.7–5.6) when comparing women without children at home to all men.

** All upper extremity disorders combined

reported, whether these covariates had confounded the association with gender could not be determined.

Two studies with data on both men and women used physical examinations to obtain MSD diagnoses (Table 3). The larger of these two studies, by Hales et al., did not show that gender was a risk factor for disorders of any part of the neck or upper extremity.[24] In contrast, the one study by Bergqvist et al. that failed to exhibit gender differences in questionnaire responses did show women to have higher prevalences for three of four diagnostic categories.[19] In that study, the occurrence of both tension neck syndrome and the group of all arm/hand diagnoses among women also appeared to be influenced by child-care duties (see below).

In the study by Bergqvist et al., both symptoms and diagnoses were reported by gender, permitting the two types of endpoints to be compared directly.[19] As already noted, differences in symptom frequencies between men and women in that study were fairly small, whereas diagnosed disorders were 1.5–10 times more frequent among women than men. As a group, women were considerably more likely than men to have their upper extremity and neck discomforts "confirmed" by a diagnosis in the corresponding region (Table 4). These data are not consistent with the idea that the difference between men and women results from a greater tendency to report symptoms by women. However, some caveats are appropriate here. First, VDU-specific data are available only for this one study; secondly, this study is the only one *not* suggesting overall differences in questionnaire data; finally, the published data allow only comparisons of group prevalences, not associations between individuals' symptoms and diagnoses.

GENDER AS AN EFFECT MODIFIER

The study by Aronsson et al. was one of few to investigate whether the effect of VDU work on MSDs differed between men and women, i.e., whether gender was an effect modifier of VDU work.[20] For neck symptoms, the male-specific odds ratios

TABLE 4.   Comparison of Prevalences of Symptoms Ascertained by Questionnaires and Diagnoses Obtained through Medical Examinations in Men and Women Employed in Video Display Unit (VDU) Work

Location	Men (n = 58)			Women (n = 189)		
	Discomforts	Diagnoses	Ratio	Discomforts	Diagnoses	Ratio
Neck	45.7%	32.8%*	0.72	54.4%	49.2%*	0.90
Shoulder	44.3%	3.3%	0.07	49.6%	14.7%	0.30
Arm/hand	28.1%	1.6%	0.06	30.4%	11.0%	0.36

* Sum of prevalences of tension neck syndromes and cervical diagnoses.
Adapted from Bergqvist U, Wolgast E, Nilsson B, Voss M: Musculoskeletal disorders among visual display terminal workers; individual, ergonomic and work organizational factors. Ergonomics 38:763–776, 1995.

were high for data entry (OR [odds ratio] = 5.5; CI [confidence interval] 2.1–14.7), data acquisition (OR = 3.8; CI 1.6–9.1), word processing (OR = 3.5; CI 1.3–2.1), and programming work (OR = 3.0; CI 1.2–7.5), compared with the reference group (mixed and varied VDU work). For shoulder problems, male data entry workers also had higher odds than male reference workers (OR = 3.4; CI 1.2–9.0) (Fig. 1). Among women, the corresponding neck and shoulder odds ratios for task type varied between 0.8 and 1.4 and were not statistically significant. Thus, gender was a strong effect modifier; men had higher risks for neck and shoulder discomforts in keyboard-intensive jobs than did women. For CAD workers no such differences were observed, nor was this effect seen for symptoms of the arm and hand region.

Figure 1 illustrates that (1) the difference in shoulder discomfort prevalences between men and women was larger in the reference group (presumably with more varied task types) than in the data entry group (with presumed more homogeneous and monotonous work); (2) women had higher prevalences than men in both task

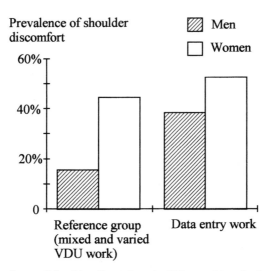

FIGURE 1.   Prevalence of shoulder discomforts in different video display unit task groups. (Adapted from Aronsson G, Bergqvist U, Almers S: Arbetsorganisation och Muskuloskeletala Besvär vid Bildskärmsarbete [Work organization and musculoskeletal discomforts in VDT work, in Swedish]. Solna, Sweden, National Institute of Working Life, 1992.)

types; and (3) the differences between the data entry and reference groups was higher for men than women. The authors speculated that "in situations with low self control of work, high time pressure, etc., the differences between men and women are fairly small—these 'external' workplace-related conditions dominate. The differences between men and women tends to increase in groups where individual (work-related) conditions are allowed to vary. In such situations, conditions outside of the workplace ('double work') may tend to 'keep' the women at a higher discomfort prevalence."

In contrast to these findings, Bergqvist et al. observed an increased risk of new hand/wrist symptoms among women with increased monotony of work over a 6-year follow-up period (risk ratio 3.1, 95% CI 1.2–7.8), whereas there was no such risk among men.[25] For neck/shoulder disorders, the only effect modification by gender was in the association with purchase of new furniture, an ambiguous finding with respect to whether the furniture was purchased before or after onset of new symptoms.

Definite conclusions are not possible, because effect modification by gender has been observed only in a few studies and not with a consistent pattern. However, if men do experience more VDU-related neck/shoulder disorders than women, even though women have a higher background risk, such a finding would have substantive and methodologic implications. The factors that cause a higher background risk in women remain to be elucidated. The selection of women only (because they have higher prevalence of disorders) in epidemiologic studies of VDU-related MSDs may actually lead to artifacts in the results, because it may limit the available exposure contrasts unnecessarily, and it should be avoided in future investigations.

INTERPRETATION OF GENDER DIFFERENCES: PHYSIOLOGIC, OCCUPATIONAL, AND SOCIOLOGICAL ISSUES

The epidemiologic evidence showed that upper extremity disorders were generally more common among women than men using VDUs occupationally. However, in the few studies that compared men and women in fairly homogeneous job groups, similar rates of MSDs were found. To the extent that there are real gender differences in work-related MSDs, their interpretation is not self-evident. Numerous factors play a role in the occurrence or reporting of these disorders.

On average, men and women differ in many aspects of physical body size and functional capacity, such as the lengths of body segments, flexibility or range of motion, and muscle strength.[26,27] These average differences may lead to a poorer fit, in general, between workstation dimensions and body size and shape for women than for men, because many workstations are "designed" for men, if they are designed at all. For example, women with a narrower shoulder width are at a greater anthropometric disadvantage when using the wider extended keyboard with a mouse.[28] It also has been hypothesized that the average difference in range of motion at the elbow—the carrying angle—may lead to more pronounced shoulder abduction and wrist ulnar deviation for women when the arms are pronated and the hands held in position over a parallel-row keyboard. However, the relevance of these anthropometric and physiologic characteristics for susceptibility to work-related MSDs remains to be examined. For most of these measures, there is a large overlap between the distributions for the two genders, i.e., despite the mean differences, many individual women are larger or stronger than many individual men.

Other physiologic factors that may affect work performance and thus possibly interact with ergonomic exposures include differences between men and women in mix of muscle fiber types (fast- and slow-twitch) and in cardiovascular endurance. Several authors have noted the potential relevance of endocrine influences, such as pregnancy, oral contraceptive use, and oophorectomy, on the occurrence of carpal tunnel syndrome. However, the evidence is inconsistent as to whether hormonal status is an important risk factor for carpal tunnel syndrome in the presence of substantial ergonomic exposures at work. These factors have not been proposed as relevant for other disorders, such as myalgia, tendon inflammation, and degenerative joint disease.

Bergqvist et al.[19] reported an increased risk of upper extremity disorders among women with occupational job demands who also had young children at home. There was no discernible difference in risk between men with and without children at home. No other evidence is available regarding the effect of household work on MSDs among VDU users. To date, there has been little formal examination of the physical or the psychosocial ergonomic features of housework in general.

Women might also experience a higher background risk of MSDs than men because of differences in level and type of psychosocial strain, both at and outside work. Jobs where women are concentrated are associated with greater psychosocial stress than men's jobs because of factors such as greater monotony, less control over the work process, less latitude for making autonomous decisions, and fewer opportunities for job modification.[4,29] In many economic sectors, women are disproportionately employed in occupations that are characterized by repetitive, low-force, manual motion patterns.[6] Similarly, in office settings, women seem to be engaged in more repetitive tasks, such as data entry, than in professional jobs with a high variety of tasks. Other sources of psychosocial strain in the workplace that may be more common or more important for women than men include responsibility to multiple supervisors, such as is found in clerical work; unpredictable, "flexible" scheduling that interferes with family responsibilities, especially caring for children; and sex discrimination and overt sexual harassment.

Medical care-seeking behavior often varies between men and women, but findings vary as to whether women and men with MSD symptoms seek care at different rates.[30-34] In occupational studies of MSDs, women have been suspected of overreporting symptoms or malingering.[35] However, there has been little formal comparison of the validity of MSD symptoms reported by male and female workers. Bergqvist et al. suggested that women VDU users were not more likely than men to report symptoms without physical examination findings.[19] However, examination methods do not necessarily provide a gold standard for validation; some types of musculoskeletal pain are difficult to diagnose with existing clinical tools. Although pain is inherently subjective, it is a legitimate entity for study and prevention. Furthermore, pain motivates the behaviors that result in costs associated with MSDs, such as seeking medical care, work absenteeism, and filing claims for compensation.

CONCLUSION

VDU work has been found to be a risk factor for upper extremity musculoskeletal disorders among women and men. Although women working with VDUs reported MSDs more frequently than men, the difference was notably less evident when men and women were compared within homogeneous job groups.

In most but not all studies comparing male and female VDU operators, the odds for neck and shoulder symptoms were about twice as high for women as for men. However, Bergqvist et al. and the SHARP report generally failed to find differences between men and women, and Burt et al. found only neck symptoms to be more prevalent.[17,19,36] Possible explanations for the discrepancies are chance, unmeasured confounding, and the fact that two of the three studies without gender differences were performed at workplaces with a high degree of routine work for all subjects.

The literature revealed limited and inconsistent evidence that ergonomic exposures in VDU work had different effects on women and men in their risk of MSDs. Data that might clarify the causes of this gender difference are sparse, either in studies of VDU users or other groups of workers. Few investigations have sought to elucidate specific factors that might explain differences in risk among VDU users, such as the types of work tasks performed by men and women or whether subjects also cared for young children at home. Data from one study permitted an analysis of whether symptoms reported by women and men were disproportionate to their findings on physical examination, and the results showed, in fact, that a higher proportion of women's symptoms appeared to be confirmed by examination, arguing against the explanation that women have a lower pain threshold or otherwise overreport symptoms.

More research is needed with regard to whether women are at higher risk of MSDs than men in jobs with the same occupational exposures. Because few epidemiologic studies have examined this question in any industry or economic sector, there is little evidence to compare with the data from office settings. In one recent study of automobile manufacturing, women workers had about a 1.5 times higher prevalence than men of upper extremity disorders, defined both by symptoms or physical examination findings.[37] However, there was substantial effect modification of ergonomic exposure by gender; women had a higher baseline prevalence than men, in the lower exposure groups, but about the same prevalence in the highest exposure group. On the other hand, after 1 year of follow-up, the cumulative incidence of new upper extremity disorders did not vary between men and women, nor did the risk associated with exposure to physical stressors.[38]

We conclude that upper extremity MSDs are exposure-related in men and women using VDUs, and there is adequate scientific knowledge regarding specific aspects of VDU work to prevent many of the MSDs. Preventive measures should not and need not be discriminatory with respect to gender.

REFERENCES

1. Bernard BP: Musculoskeletal Disorders and Workplace Factors: A Critical Review of Epidemiologic Evidence for Work-related Musculoskeletal Disorders of the Neck, Upper Extremity, and Low Back. Pub. No. 97-141. Cincinnati, National Institute for Occupational Safety and Health, 1997.
2. Punnett L, Bergqvist U: Visual Display Unit Work and Upper Extremity Musculoskeletal Disorders: A Review of Epidemiologic Findings. Solna, Sweden, National Institute of Working Life, 1997.
3. Mergler D: Adjusting for gender differences in occupational health studies. In Messing K, Neis B, Dumais L (eds): Invisible Issues in Women's Occupational Health. Charlottetown, Canada, Gynergy Books, 1995, pp 236–251.
4. Karasek RA, Theorell T: Healthy Work. Stress, Productivity and the Reconstruction of Working Life. New York, Basic Books, 1990.
5. Messing K, Dumais L, Courville J, et al: Evaluation of exposure data from men and women with the same job title. J Occup Med 36:913–917, 1994.
6. Silverstein BA, Fine LJ, Armstrong TJ: Hand wrist cumulative trauma disorders in industry. Br J Ind Med 43:779–784, 1986.
7. Silverstein BA, Fine LJ, Armstrong TJ: Occupational factors and carpal tunnel syndrome. Am J Ind Med 11:343–358, 1987.
8. Loscocco KA, Spitze G: Working conditions, social support and the well-being of female and male factory workers. J Health Soc Behav 31:313–327, 1990.
9. Mergler D, Brabant C, Vézina N, Messing K: The weaker sex? Men in women's working conditions report similar health symptoms. J Occup Med 29:417–421, 1987.

10. National Research Council: Video Displays, Work and Vision: Panel on Impact of Video Viewing on Vision of Workers. Washington, DC, National Academy Press, 1983.
11. Bongers PM, de Winter CR, Kompier MAJ, Hildebrandt VH: Psychosocial factors at work and musculoskeletal disease. Scand J Work Environ Health 19:297–312, 1993.
12. Gerr F, Marcus M, Ortiz DJ: Methodological limitations in the study of video display terminal use and upper extremity musculoskeletal disorders. Am J Ind Med 29:649–656, 1996.
13. Faucett J, Rempel D: VDT-related musculoskeletal symptoms: Interactions between work posture and psychosocial work factors. Am J Ind Med 26:597–612, 1994.
14. Oxenburgh MS: Musculoskeletal injuries occurring in word processing operators. In Stevenson M (ed): Readings in RSI: The Ergonomic Approach to Repetition Strain Injuries. Kensington, Australia, New South Wales University Press, 1987, pp 91–95.
15. Ferreira JM, Conceicao GM, Saldiva PH: Work organization is significantly associated with upper extremity musculoskeletal disorders among employees engaged in interactive computer-telephone tasks of an international bank subsidiary in Sao Paulo, Brazil. Am J Ind Med 31:468–473, 1997.
16. Evans J: Women, men, VDU work and health: A questionnaire survey of British VDU operators. Work Stress 1:271–283, 1987.
17. Safety and Health Assessment & Research For Prevention: Cumulative Trauma Disorders in Claims Follow-up Study. Olympia, WA, Washington State Department of Labor and Industries, 1993.
18. Polanyi MFD, Cole DC, Beaton DE, et al: Upper limb work-related musculoskeletal disorders among newspaper employees: Cross-sectional survey results. Am J Ind Med 32:620–628, 1997.
19. Bergqvist U, Wolgast E, Nilsson B, Voss M: Musculoskeletal disorders among visual display terminal workers; individual, ergonomic and work organizational factors. Ergonomics 38:763–776, 1995.
20. Aronsson G, Bergqvist U, Almers S: Arbetsorganisation och Muskuloskeletala Besvär vid Bildskärmsarbete (Work organization and musculoskeletal discomforts in VDT work, in Swedish). Solna, Sweden, National Institute of Working Life, 1992.
21. Bernard BP, Sauter S, Fine LJ, et al: Job task and psychosocial risk factors for work-related musculoskeletal disorders among newspaper employees. Scand J Work Environ Health 20:417–426, 1994.
22. Knave B, Wibom R, Voss M, et al: Work with video display terminals among office employees. I. Subjective symptoms and discomfort. Scand J Work Environ Health 11:457–466, 1985.
23. Hales TR, Sauter SL, Peterson MR, et al: Health Hazard Evaluation Report. U.S. West Communications, Phoenix AZ, Minneapolis/St Paul MN, Denver CO. Cincinnati, National Institute for Occupational Safety and Health, 1992, HETA 82-299-2230.
24. Hales TR, Sauter SL, Peterson MR, et al: Musculoskeletal disorders among visual display terminal users in a telecommunications company. Ergonomics 37:1603–1621, 1994.
25. Bergqvist U: Visual display terminal work—a perspective on long-term changes and discomforts. Int J Ind Ergon 16:201–209, 1995.
26. Chaffin DB, Andersson GBJ: Occupational Biomechanics. New York, Wiley & Sons, 1991.
27. Mital A, Kumar S: Human muscle strength definitions, measurement, and usage: part II—The scientific basis (knowledge base) for the guide. Int J Ind Ergon 22:123–144, 1998.
28. Karlqvist L: Assessment of Physical Work Load at Visual Display Unit Workstations. Ergonomic Applications and Gender Aspects. Solna, Sweden, National Institute of Working Life, 1997.
29. Hall EM: Women's Work: An Inquiry into the Health Effects of Invisible and Visible Labor. Stockholm, Karolinska Institute, 1990.
30. Bush FM, Harkins SW, Harrington WG, Price DD: Analysis of gender effects on pain perception and symptom presentation in temporomandibular pain. Pain 53:73–80, 1993.
31. Carey T, Evans A, Hadler N, et al: Acute severe low back pain: A population-based study of prevalence and care-seeking. Spine 21:339–344, 1996.
32. Harreby M, Kjer J, Hesselsoe G, Neergaard K: Epidemiological aspects and risk factors for low back pain in 38-year-old men and women: A 25-year prospective cohort study of 640 school children. Eur Spine J 5:312–318, 1996.
33. Hurwitz EL, Morgenstern H: The effects of comorbidity and other factors on medical versus chiropractic care for back problems. Spine 22:2254–2263, 1997.
34. Von Korff M, Wagner EH, Dworkin SF, Saunders KW: Chronic pain and use of ambulatory health care. Psychosom Med 53:61–79, 1991.
35. Cleland L: "RSI": A model of social iatrogenesis. Med J Aust 147:236–239, 1987.
36. Burt S, Hornung R, Fine LJ: Health Hazard Evaluation Report. Newsday Inc., Melville, NY. Cincinnati, National Institute for Occupational Safety and Health, 1990, HETA 89-250-2046.
37. Punnett L: Upper extremity disorders among male and female automotive manufacturing workers. Proceedings of the 13 Triennial Congress of the International Ergonomics Association, Tampere, Finland, 1997, pp 512–514.

38. Punnett L: Comparison of Analytic Methods for a Follow-up Study of Upper Extremity Disorders PREMUS-ISEOH 98. Helsinki, Finnish Institute of Occupational Health, 1998.

39. Bosi Ferraz M, Frumkin H, Helfenstein M, et al: Upper-extremity musculoskeletal disorders in keyboard operators in Brazil: A cross-sectional study. Int J Occup Environ Health 1:239–244, 1995.

ROBERT F. BETTENDORF

A LOW-COST, EFFECTIVE APPROACH TO OFFICE ERGONOMICS

From The Institute for Office
  Ergonomics, Inc.
Manchester Center, Vermont

Reprint requests to:
Robert F. Bettendorf
The Institute for Office Ergonomics,
  Inc.
River Road
P.O. Box 1267
Manchester Center, VT 05255

Office workers experience surprisingly high levels of on-the-job discomfort. The most common complaints are headaches, eye strain, and neck, shoulder, arm, hand, and back pain. Workers commonly do not understand that their discomforts may be caused by the set-up of their workstations and their working postures. People might complain that their back always hurts at the end of the day because they have back problems, but they rarely ascribe their symptoms to the way their chair is adjusted.

These discomforts exist even in offices that have the latest ergonomic furniture, because the personal computer (PC) is installed improperly or the furniture is not adjusted to fit the user. This chapter outlines the discomforts normally associated with office work, their potential causes, and how they can be reduced or prevented at low cost or no cost before they become more serious problems. The emphasis is on how to maximize the ergonomic suitability of existing furniture, lighting, and PCs. Experience has shown that extensive replacement of existing facilities and equipment is costly and unnecessary in most situations.

MUSCULOSKELETAL PROBLEMS IN THE OFFICE ENVIRONMENT

Like any other new issue that management faces, the right first step is to determine the real nature of the problem. Clinical conditions such as carpal tunnel syndrome and upper extremity musculoskeletal disorders sometimes occur in office workers, but on-the-job discomforts are much more prevalent.

The United States Bureau of Labor Statistics (BLS) reports yearly on the number of newly

TABLE 1.   Types of Complaints Voiced by Office Workers during
an Ergonomics Evaluation*

Type of Complaint	Number of Complaints	% Total Employees
Headache/eye strain	119	25%
Neck and shoulder	83	17%
Backache	54	11%
Wrist, arm, hand	14	3%
Leg	4	1%
Total	274	

* Of 475 workers who were surveyed, 173 voiced complaints.

reported occupational injuries and illness in private industry. According to the latest statistics, in 1996, there were 11,266 repeated trauma cases with a reported association between typing or key entry tasks and time off from work.[4] Although this number is small, the cases are expensive to resolve and require more time off than typical occupational injuries. The BLS also reports on the median days away from work, a key measure of severity. In 1996, the median time away from work was 5 days for all injuries and illnesses and 17 days for repetitive motion injuries.

Despite the low number of musculoskeletal disorders in most office settings, worker discomfort is common. A typical example of the level of office worker discomfort comes from interviews conducted at the headquarters of the Hoechst Celanese Corporation, a chemical and pharmaceutical manufacturer based in Somerville, New Jersey.[1] In 1991, Hoechst implemented an office ergonomics program even though the company's administrative, professional, and secretarial employees were not raising any health concerns. At total of 475 individual PC workstation evaluations were performed. During the evaluation, 173 (36%) employees acknowledged having experienced on-the-job discomforts such as headaches, neck aches, or other problems (Table 1).

Eighteen employees described their discomfort as serious, constant, frequent, or severe or stated that they were being treated for them by a doctor or a chiropractor.

The largest number of complaints were vision-related: headaches and eye strain described as "tired eyes," "itchy eyes," and "eye discomfort." This high percentage is typical when the work areas are too bright.

The low number of wrist, arm, or hand discomforts may be surprising but was typical of most office environments prior to the widespread use of pointing devices such as a computer mouse.

Table 2 contrasts these results with symptom surveys conducted at five newspapers and two government agencies. At Hoechst, the levels of complaints were far lower than in all the other surveys. Although there were some methodology differences in the surveys and the level of installed ergonomics was probably different, this would not explain the eightfold to seventeenfold increase in hand and wrist complaints. Once probable explanation is that ergonomic working conditions were not an issue between employees and management at Hoechst, but they were a major issue in the newspaper industry. The ergonomic issues in four of the five other surveyed groups were so severe that NIOSH was asked to perform health hazard evaluations of the working environment and conditions.

AN OFFICE ERGONOMICS PROGRAM

The primary objective of an office ergonomics program is to reduce on-the-job discomforts before employees require time off from work, medical treatment, or

TABLE 2. Surveys of Office Workers' Symptoms

Organization	Hoechst Celanese Corporation	Three Newspapers*	Social Security Office, Boston	Social Security Office, Fort Lauderdale, Florida	Newsday	Los Angeles Times
Date	1991–1992	1991–1992	1993	1993	1990	1990
Population	475	200	31	77	834	825
Conducted by	IOE	University of Iowa	NIOSH	NIOSH	NIOSH	NIOSH
Symptoms Reported						
Neck	17%	43%	23%	53%	17%	26%
Shoulder		L 21% R 23%	13%	44%	11%	17%
Elbow and Forearm	1%	L 8% R 6%	19%	21%	13%	10%
Hand/wrist	2%	L 20% R 22%	16%	35%	23%	22%
Back Upper back	11%	26%	23%	38%		
Lower back		43%				
Headaches and eye complaints	25%					

* Cedar Rapids Gazette, Peoria Journal, Quail City Times
IOE = The Institute for Office Ergonomics, Inc., Manchester Center, Vermont; NIOSH = National Institute for Occupational Safety and Health; L = left; R = right

workers' compensation benefits. Avoiding one large workers' compensation claim might pay for an ergonomics program.

Great strides have been made in bringing overall medical and workers' compensation costs under control, but they are still significant. According to U.S. Chamber of Commerce's *Employee Benefits 1997 Edition*, the average employer expenditure for medical insurance, sick leave, and short- and long-term disability was $3,061. The National Council on Compensation Insurance reports that the average workers' compensation claim for indemnity and medical was $17,900 in 1995.[3] A recent report by the General Accounting Office confirms that ergonomics programs can positively affect the number of injuries and illnesses, lost and restricted workdays, and the cost of claims related to musculoskeletal disorders.[5] The report shows that American Express reduced its total workers' compensation costs by 80% and the average cost of musculoskeletal-related claims from $9,123 to $1,685 with its office ergonomics program.

The second objective is to demonstrate management's concern for the health and well being of its employees. As the labor market tightens, a good working environment will help attract and keep good employees. An ergonomics program will reduce on-the-job discomfort and fatigue, thereby improving the quality of the office process with positive effects on productivity and error rates.

The factors that cause or contribute to fatigue, discomfort, and pain in an office workplace are well known, and they exist to some degree in most offices. They include working in awkward postures, typing or using a mouse with the wrists in a nonneutral posture, repeatedly twisting the neck, using a chair that does not fit properly, working under poor lighting conditions, having improper vision correction, and having insufficient rest and recovery time.

The negative effect of these ergonomic risk factors can be reduced or eliminated by a program that:

- Ensures that workstations are set up properly and have a correct lighting environment,
- Trains employees how to avoid common musculoskeletal and visual problems, and
- Encourages the reporting of ergonomic problems so that they can be addressed.

AN OFFICE ERGONOMICS PRIMER

Achieving proper workstation organization and the right lighting environment and correcting any vision deficiencies are necessary to avoid pain and discomfort. Primers on the right way to set up a PC workstation and on lighting and vision follow. They are written in the second person so that they can be used to counsel employees on ergonomics and become the script for an ergonomics training program.

A Personal Computer Workstation

The key to ergonomically correct PC work is to be seated comfortably, with your back well supported and your feet on the floor. The way you organize the other elements of your workstation can help you do your job more effectively and comfortably. You should avoid excessive reaches. Keep the telephone, calculator, and other frequently used items within an arm's length of your primary working position.

When you type, your forearms should be parallel to the floor with the wrists in a neutral posture. Avoid bending your wrists. Typing with the wrists flexed forward like a praying mantis or extended as if playing a piano while standing will put unnecessary strains on your tendons and can lead to discomfort.

To achieve the right wrist posture, raise or lower your chair until your forearms are parallel to the floor and the wrists are in the neutral position. Your elbows should be at the same height as the home or center row of the keyboard. This neutral posture also can be achieved by raising or lowering the typing work surface or by using a keyboard tray that can be raised or lowered.

Some chairs are raised or lowered by twisting the seat back while restraining the base with your foot; these chairs may need to be readjusted periodically. To adjust chairs with a pneumatic mechanism, sit on the chair and press the lever under the seat to lower it completely. Raise your body to the right height while pressing the lever. The chair will raise and lock in position when your body stops it.

If your feet are not flat on the floor when your arms are in the correct position, you should be using a footrest.

Your chair should support your back while you are typing. Although changing your position periodically is recommended, do not lean forward for extended periods. Lack of back support causes back pain. Some chairs allow you to adjust the backrest to improve your comfort and back support. Raise or lower it until the lumbar support fits into the small of your back. In some cases, a back support cushion may help.

If your chair is broken, uncomfortable, or does not provide proper back support, it may require some adjustment or repair. Sometimes a new or swapped chair is required to make sure that your chair is the proper size.

The placement of your PC on the workstation is critical. The monitor and keyboard should be directly in front of you to avoid excessive neck movements. Placing the monitor to the side can sometimes cause a pain in the neck.

The top of the monitor's case should be at or slightly below eye level. If you look straight ahead and see the top section or the middle of the screen, the monitor is too high. Even this slight elevation will cause you to tilt your head upward, which frequently leads to neck and shoulder pain. A monitor that is installed on top of the PC control unit is usually too high. To lower it, place the control unit on the side or under your desk. A vertical stand will properly support the control unit while it is on the floor.

A PC can be correctly installed on a narrow surface by using a keyboard drawer, tray, or caddy. Avoid sitting on or crossing your legs while typing. Clean out the area under your workstation so that your feet do not trip over boxes or your wastepaper basket.

If your job requires input from source documents, use a copy holder. The holder should be installed so that the copy is next to and at the same height as the monitor. This will reduce the amount of eye and neck movement necessary to go back and forth between the display screen and the source documents.

If you type while using the telephone, use a head set. Cradling the phone between your ear and shoulder is not comfortable and makes it difficult to work.

If you develop pain or discomfort in the upper arm or shoulder while using the mouse, it is probably due to stretching or reaching to use the mouse. Move the mouse to either side of and directly next to the keyboard.

Finger and hand discomfort can be caused by a mouse that does not fit your hand properly or if you use too much force. Mice come come in different sizes; make sure that yours feels comfortable and allows you to use it without awkward finger postures. Hold the mouse lightly and push the buttons with a minimum of force. You should never need to lift the mouse off the mouse pad to move the cursor across or down the screen. If you do, increase the mouse tracking speed. If necessary, you also can change the double click speed. Keyboard commands can be used in place of mouse functions. Also, occasionally change the hand with which you use the mouse.

Workloads without time for rest and recovery can lead to fatigue and discomfort. Make sure that you take your lunch and scheduled breaks. If you begin to feel any pain or discomfort, stop and take a short break. Stretch and walk around for a little bit to rest your tired muscles. Sometimes these mini-breaks are all you need to prevent or reduce on-the-job discomforts. Another approach is to intersperse demanding computer work or other repetitive tasks with other work.

Lighting and Vision

Many PC users experience occasional headaches, eye strain, tired eyes, or other visually related discomforts. Improper lighting, reflections or glare on the monitor's screen, dirty screens, or improperly corrected vision can cause eye discomforts and headaches.

The first step in reducing risk factors is to look at the display. You should not see reflections from ceiling lights, credenza lights, or windows; reflections can cause eye discomfort and headaches. To eliminate reflections:
- Tilt your monitor forward to eliminate the source of glare.
- Turn off unnecessary credenza lights, particularly those above the monitor or within your field of vision.

- If possible, reposition the keyboard and monitor so they are perpendicular to the windows. You should neither face the windows nor have them directly behind you while working on the PC.
- Close the window blinds when the sun is reflecting or shining directly on the monitor.
- If you still have glare on the screen, install a glare screen.

Keep the monitor's screen clean using a wipe or a glass cleaner. Also, vary the brightness and contrast controls until the image is clear and the most pleasing to your eyes.

If the above suggestions do not eliminate headaches and eye discomfort, remove half of the fluorescent lights in the existing fixtures and turn off unnecessary credenza lights. Offices are frequently lit well above recommended levels.

Many contact lens wearers do not blink often enough. Staring at the screen may dry out your eyes and cause temporary irritation. Blink more frequently to keep your eyes moist.

When your eyes get tired, periodically look up and focus on a distant object, such as a clock or a picture on the wall.

Wearers of bifocals may experience neck discomfort from raising their chin to peer out of the bottom of their glasses while reading the screen. Lowering the monitor or the worksurface might help. If not, continuous focal-length glasses or glasses designed for PC use may be the answer.

If these suggestions do not work, consult your eye care specialist. Almost one of three adults either needs glasses or needs a change in their prescription. An improper prescription can cause eye discomfort and fatigue. The use of PCs does present some special vision requirements. Eyeglasses are normally set for a reading of 12–14 inches, but the PC monitor is probably 20–28 inches or more from your eyes. Measure the distance from your eyes to the center of the screen so that the right glasses for PC work can be prescribed for you.

AN IMPLEMENTATION APPROACH

This section describes a short-term plan to resolve ergonomics problems at no or low cost and a longer-term plan to improve the ergonomic capabilities of your existing facilities. The following steps are recommended:

- Do an ergonomic walk-through
- Decide on the use of a consultant
- Form an ergonomics committee
- Develop a plan
- Obtain management commitment
- Conduct staff and supervisor training
- Develop an ergonomic purchasing strategy

An Ergonomic Walk-Through

Using the prior sections as a guide, walk through enough of your departments to develop a feel for whether the chairs and workstations are set up and being used properly. Observe the postures of the PC users. Ask a few employees if they know how to adjust their chairs. If the worksurfaces are adjustable, how many have been raised or lowered? Most workstations are 29–30 inches high, but a study shows that 25–27 inches is the best height for most workers in the U.S.[2] How many ergonomic accessories are being used? Are employees who need to type while talking on the phone using a head set? Are document holders used?

Sit at a few workstations to determine if there is glare on the screen. Are there any annoying light sources in your field of vision? See how many people are squinting when they read the screen or are perched on the edge of the chair because they cannot read the characters when they sit back.

Ask some employees if they have discomforts at the end of the day. If they say no, prompt them by asking again if they ever have any neck pain, headaches, or back pain. Keep an informal scorecard and compare it to the discomfort surveys shown in Table 2.

Table 3 summarizes the results of 475 individual evaluations conducted at Hoechst Celanese. More than 90% of the evaluations resulted in some recommendation. About half of the workstations were set up incorrectly, and more than half had too much ambient light or glare on the screen. Even though the workstations were adjustable, almost all of them were set at 29 inches high. One third of them need to be lowered. About 10% of the chairs needed to be repaired. Another 10% did not provide proper back support or had 19-inch seat pans, which were too deep for the users. Few workstations or video display terminal (VDT) tables needed to be replaced or modified, but many ergonomic accessories were needed.

TABLE 3. Ergonomic Evaluation Results at Hoechst Celanese Corporation

	Number	Percent
Individual ergonomic evaluations completed	475	
Some changes recommended	443	93%
No changes needed	32	7%
Summary of recommendations		
Ergonomic accessories recommended	467	
Lighting/screen glare related	242	51%
PC set up improperly	223	47%
Height of work surface to be changed	158	33%
Chair repair, replacement, or swap		
Chair broken	45	
Improper back support	23	
Seat pan too deep	34	
Total	102	21%
Workstation recommendations		
New furniture needed	5	
New furniture possibly needed	3	
Add a corner unit	9	
New VDT table needed	11	
Replace VDT table	4	
Total	32	7%
Ergonomic accessories recommended		
Keyboard caddies	75	
Keyboard drawers	18	
Articulating keyboard trays	6	
Vertical CPU stands	198	
Antiglare filters	56	
Document holders	74	
Footrests	8	
Telephone headsets	5	
Phone cradles	6	
Floor mats	3	
Longer cables	5	
Task lamps	13	
Total	467	

PC = personal computer; VDT = video display terminal; CPU = central processing unit

A properly conducted walk-through should define the extent of the ergonomic problems, give you some idea of the cost to correct them, and help ensure that your program is properly targeted. The next two steps can be undertaken in the sequence that seems best to you.

The Consultant's Role

A consultant's expertise can be helpful in the early phases of a program's development. You should first decide if you have time to define the program and make it happen. The right consultant can facilitate the process, and his fees may be covered by eliminating unnecessary purchases of ergonomic furniture and accessories. Ergonomic self-sufficiency should be your objective.

The Ergonomics Committee

Many companies have used an ergonomics committee to reach consensus on the need for ergonomic improvements. The committee can serve as a forum to identify and resolve problems and to obtain the necessary line and staff commitments. It can also be the platform from which to secure management support. The membership is critical to the success of the committee and the ergonomics program. It should include representatives from human resources, the medical department, facilities, information systems, administration, and line management.

Representation from information systems is important, because that is the group that usually chooses new PCs and also may be responsible to set new PCs. If they order monitors without antiglare treatment, the number of headaches and eye complaints will increase, and antiglare screens will need to be purchased at $80 to $120 each.

Developing a Plan

Using the results of the walk-through, the ergonomics committee and any consultants develop a plan, decide on the level of activity for each program element, and make sure that all the necessary implementation commitments are in place and any remaining issues defined.

Before seeking approval for the plan, anticipate the questions and objections that management might ask. You should be able to answer three important questions:
• Why do we need to do this?
• What will it cost?
• What do we expect to get from this?

Most management will readily agree to replace a broken chair, buy a document holder, or train employees how to derive ergonomic benefits from the existing chairs and furniture. Their concern is that an ergonomics program might result in extensive replacement of chairs, workstations, or ceiling luminaries. The walk-through and the ergonomic purchasing strategy (described below) should provide enough information to quell any fears on this point. If not, a consultant can be sought to provide an expert opinion on how to improve the ergonomic suitability of the existing facilities without large expenditures.

Management Commitment

Your objective should be to secure senior management support for the program and the resources required to conduct the training, purchase ergonomic accessories, and to fund modest other purchases to resolve specific situations in which a new workstation or chair may be required. You should also secure the support for the future ergonomic purchases strategy and resolve any other issues. A letter pledging support for the program from senior management to the line and staff management can be helpful in smoothing the implementation phase.

Staff and Supervisory Training

Ergonomic training should be conducted for supervisors and employees. The supervisors should be trained because they are probably PC users and need to understand and support the ergonomics program.

The following eight points outline an agenda for an hour-long office ergonomics training program. The tone should be upbeat and focus on how to improve on-the-job comfort rather than how to avoid a cumulative trauma disorder.

1. Program introduction: objectives, management commitment, and agenda.
2. Ergonomic video: several videos are available from vendors. Choose one that has the right message and fits with your corporate culture.
3. Review the right way to set up a PC workstation through slides of good and bad PC set-ups, or use a PC, ergonomic chair, and workstation for a demonstration. The section of this chapter, A Personal Computer Workstation, can be used as a guide.
4. Emphasize the common factors that contribute to office discomforts:
   Neck aches—monitor too high or in wrong location.
   Back aches—chair fit, adjustment, lack of lumbar support, need for glasses.
   Hand pain while using the mouse—mouse fit or work style.
   Upper arm pain while using the mouse—mouse location.
   Tired eyes and headaches—lighting, screen glare, glare sources, need for
       new glasses.
   Discuss the need for rest breaks.
5. Discuss vision and lighting using the section in this chapter on these subjects as a guide.
6. Encourage the reporting of any ergonomic discomforts so that problems can be addressed.
7. Offer to help individuals change their workstations if they cannot do it themselves.
8. Identify how to seek help, i.e., to obtain an ergonomic accessory, a longer printer or telephone cable, or to remove tubes in the ceiling fixtures.

Ergonomics training programs are also available from ergonomic suppliers. However, because many of them do not cover vision and lighting adequately, you may have to add information on this important subject.

An Ergonomic Purchasing Strategy

Your overall objective should be to maximize the ergonomic capabilities of existing furniture and lighting and to then gradually improve the ergonomic suitability of the facilities over time through new purchases as you expand or renovate.

As part of this strategy, set guidelines for all future ergonomic purchases. Pick the ergonomic accessories that work in your situations and make them easily available to employees. Do not buy one of anything for everybody except mouse pads. Also, do not set up a procedure by which four people would need to approve the purchase of an inexpensive accessory. It is usually more difficult to get people to use the accessories than it is to deal with the one or two who may want everything regardless of whether they need it. Avoid any product that claims, for instance, that it will "prevent carpal tunnel syndrome." Ask for the supporting evidence. Chances are that it does not exist or is weak.

Pick a furniture dealer who either understands ergonomics or can provide expert support from the manufacturer or a consultant. Almost all of the common ergonomic problems of existing workstations can be improved at low cost. If your dealer cannot help, search for one who can.

For new purchases, buy workstations with adjustable work surfaces. If they are used on more than shift, they should be easily adjustable.

Buy quality ergonomic chairs with good lumbar support and ergonomic options such as adjustable backrests and armrests. Buy more than one size so the chairs can properly fit employees of various sizes. Resist the notion that it is acceptable to spend more for a chair for a manager who rarely uses it but much less for a chair for a worker who spends most of the day in it.

Tie in the purchasing strategy with the information systems strategy. Make sure that equipment has good ergonomic capabilities and will fit on your current workstations.

CONCLUSION

Discomfort levels in most offices are surprisingly high. Their causes and ways to reduce or eliminate them are well known. Although the subject of ergonomics may be intimidating to lay persons, many feel that office ergonomics is really "informed common sense." Following the suggestions in this chapter can have a positive effect on employee morale, job satisfaction, and well being. The benefits can be achieved with some effort while avoiding expensive purchases.

REFERENCES

1. Hoechst Celanese: Office Ergonomic Solutions: Six Case Studies. Alexandria, VA, Center for Office Technology, 1994.
2. Konrad K: Population Segment Accommodation for Keyboard Entry at Various Workstations. The Knoll Group, 1992.
3. NCCI 1997 Issues Report. Boca Raton, FL, National Council on Compensation Insurance, 1997.
4. NIOSH: Health Hazard Evaluation Report: Los Angeles Times, Los Angeles, California. Cincinnati, Ohio, U.S. Department of Health and Human Services, Public Health Services, Centers for Disease Control, National Institute for Occupational Safety and Health, Report No. HETA 90-013-2277, 1993.
5. NIOSH: Health Hazard Evaluation Report: Newsday, Inc., Melville, NY. Cincinnati, Ohio, U.S. Department of Health and Human Services, Public Health Services, Centers for Disease Control, National Institute for Occupational Safety and Health, Report No. HETA 89-250-2046, 1990.
6. NIOSH: Health Hazard Evaluation Report: Social Security Administration Teleservice Centers, Boston, Massachuesetts & Fort Lauderdale, Florida. Cincinnati, Ohio, U.S. Department of Health and Human Services, Public Health Services, Centers for Disease Control, National Institute for Occupational Safety and Health, Report No. HETA 92-0382-2450, 1994.
7. United States Department of Labor, Bureau of Labor Statistics: Lost-Worktime Injuries and Illnesses: Characteristics and Resulting Time Away from Work, 1996. Washington, DC, BLS, 1998, USDL-98-157.
8. United States General Accounting Office: Worker Protection, Private Sector Ergonomic Programs Yield Positive Results. Washington, DC, GAO, 1997. GAO/HEHS-97-163.
9. The University of Iowa: Multi-Site Newspaper Study, Results Phase I, 1991. The University of Iowa, Iowa City, 1992.

IVAN G. MOST, ScD

PSYCHOSOCIAL ELEMENTS IN THE WORK ENVIRONMENT OF A LARGE CALL CENTER OPERATION

From Strategic Occupational
  Health Management, Inc.
Cape Elizabeth, Maine

Reprint requests to:
Ivan G. Most
Strategic Occupational Health
  Management, Inc.
58 Brentwood Road
Cape Elizabeth, ME 04107

Anyone who uses the telephone to make a hotel reservation or order merchandise is interacting with a call center. Call center workers are becoming more numerous as technology changes the way commerce is undertaken worldwide. They provide critical customer interface for direct sales, marketing, and customer service. The nature of this work combines some of the elements of machine-paced manufacturing jobs with the psychosocial strain of the office environment.

To better understand musculoskeletal injuries among customer service employees at its call centers, a large catalog retailer employed this author, an engineer working in the area of occupational health, to investigate some of the psychosocial factors in place that prevent early detection of injuries. This work was undertaken with the assistance of the ergonomics and safety coordinator for the customer satisfaction department of the company. Call center employees were surveyed to better understand some of the psychosocial factors that affect their health.

As much as 80% of the company's business is transacted through catalog sales, mostly at two call centers. The company employs about 5,000 workers, nearly 1,000 of whom work in call center operations. In the mid to late 1980s, employees experienced a rising incidence of cumulative trauma disorders (CTDs) predominantly in the back and upper extremities. Even though many physical changes were undertaken to better fit the workstation to the employee, the company recognized that to successfully address the increase in CTDs a macro-ergonomic approach was required.

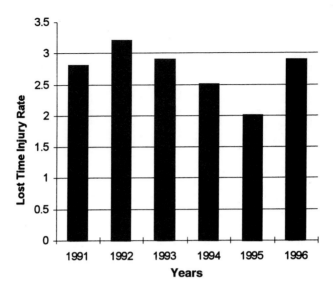

FIGURE 1. Lost-time injury rates based on 100 full-time employees in the customer satisfaction department.

The work already undertaken at the company to prevent musculoskeletal injuries included: worksite analysis, worksite modification, an ergonomics representative program to provide trained personnel onsite to adjust workstations, scheduled stretch breaks, and postoffer health inquiry, including anthropometric measures to properly fit employees to workstations. However, it was believed that biomechanical or physiologic approaches alone could not explain the cause of the increase in CTDs. Many other factors, including work organization and work systems design, needed to be addressed. The actual lost-time experience for the customer satisfaction department, which includes the call centers, is show in Figure 1. The injury rate showed a downward trend from 1992 to 1995 but started to increase in 1996. The underlying cause of the increase may not be explained by physical ergonomic stressors alone.

Ergonomic interventions are more effective when psychosocial aspects of the jobs are evaluated. Formalized job descriptions often limit the individual's decision-making responsibility; these jobs can be classified as high demand and low control. Karasek and Theorell have noted that individuals employed in these types of jobs have an increased incidence of heart disease.[6]

The employees in the call centers work as customer service representatives or order representatives. The customer service representatives generally are permanent employees, and the order representatives are temporary employees hired for particularly busy periods.

This chapter discusses work that was undertaken in 1997 and 1998 to better understand the working environment at the call centers and to determine the effect of late reporting of injury on the long-term health of workers.

BACKGROUND LITERATURE

Combining the principles of total quality management (TQM) and ergonomics was a natural step for this company because of its tradition of quality customer service and products. TQM at the company is based on five principles[6]:

1. Focus on customer needs
2. Top management support
3. Employee involvement
4. Effective measurement
5. Continuous improvement

These principles were reinforced by research by this author that explored the following primary hypotheses:[11]

- Workplace organization influences the success of health and safety programs.
- Management commitment is necessary to successfully implement new regulatory policy.
- Government sanctions can affect health and safety program implementation.

Management commitment and employee involvement, key elements of the company TQM program, also were determined to have an important role in the success of health and safety programs at the companies studied in this research.[11]

A review of relevant literature was undertaken to provide guidance in the conduct of the employee survey. One of the key issues that was investigated was the effect of early diagnosis of injury on the long-term rehabilitation of employees. Early detection was assumed to be the correct approach.

Psychosocial Effects

A literature search was conducted using the Medline data set of 3,600 medical and health journals as a primary resource and, secondarily, articles used in doctoral thesis research by this author.

A National Institute for Occupational Safety and Health report was reviewed[12] (Table 1). There were seven key psychosocial factors that indicated upper extremity musculoskeletal injury and symptoms. In addition, a recent British study of government workers showed a higher incidence (odds ratio 1.5) of coronary heart disease (CHD) among workers of lower grade than among managerial workers.[9] This supports the demand control model by Karasek and Theorell in which workers with more decision-making latitude experience a lower incidence of coronary heart disease.

Both of these studies reinforced the importance of psychosocial factors as a potential cause of employee injury. The influence of workplace organization on the incidence of occupational disease also is important.

TABLE 1. Summary of Study* of Communication Workers at US West Communications

Psychosocial Variables Associated with Upper Extremity Musculoskeletal Disorders	Psychosocial Variables Associated with the Degree of Upper Extremity Symptoms	Electronic Monitoring Systems Affecting Degree of Symptoms
Fear of being replaced by computer	All issues described in left column	Caused less socializing with employees
Jobs that require a variety of tasks	Uncertainty about one's job future	Rarely helped work performance and motivation
Increasing work pressure	Lack of coworker support	Caused more supervisor complaints regarding work performance
Lack of production standard	Lack of supervisor's support	
Lack of job diversity with little decision-making opportunity		Closely monitored their work quality
High information-processing demands		Caused more work
Surges in workload		

* HETA 89-299-2230

Workplace Organization

Many aspects of workplace organization were important to this author's study of the catalog retailer. Some prior studies considered the environmental climate in an organization and the elements of climate that define the effectiveness of a group of people and their ability to change. The research for the retailer also considered the effect of organizational structure on employee health.

Corporations organize individuals to accomplish various tasks.[2] According to Arygis, formal workplace organization is characterized by task (work) specialization, chain of command, unity of direction, and span of control (no more than five or six subordinates).[2]

Formal organizations create certain demands on individuals, which were organized by Arygis as propositions:[2]

Proposition 1: There is a lack of congruency between the needs of healthy individuals and the demands of the (initial) formal organization. (This creates a disturbance between the individual and the organization.)

Proposition 2: The result of this disturbance for individuals is frustration, short time perspective, and conflict.

Proposition 3: Under certain conditions, the degree of frustration, failure, short time perspective, and conflict will tend to increase.

Proposition 4: The nature of the formal principles of organization cause the subordinates at any given level to experience competition, rivalry, intersubordinate hostility, and to develop a focus toward the parts rather than the whole. (Tension then develops between the needs of the organization and the needs of the individuals.)

Arygis reports that some individuals note that this tension is beyond their control and coping with it requires energy to be used in the form of maintaining defenses, which tends to make individuals less productive.

In his discussion of organizational learning, Senge noted that thinking about the big picture instead of the parts is a first step in developing a "learning organization."[15] While system thinking is a major element in the learning organization and integrates many of the other elements, a shift of mind or cultural change is ultimately required to successfully develop a learning organization.

Policymakers often focus on eliminating symptoms of problems, thus producing short-term benefit but, as a result, long-term malaise. In developing a shared vision of an organization, attitudes vary from total commitment to noncompliance and apathy.

Gouldner observed that organizations fall into three types: mock, representative, and punishment-centered.[4] In summarizing the defining characteristics of each organization, Gouldner looked at factors such as the following:
- Who usually initiates the rules?
- Whose values usually legitimate the rules?
- What effects do rules have on the status of participants?
- Whose values are violated by the rules?
- What are standard explanations of deviation from rules?

Table 2 describes Gouldner's summary of the different types of organizations' response to these questions.

Moran and Volkwein developed another definition of organizational climate that treats employee perceptions: "Organizational climate is a relatively enduring characteristic of an organization which distinguishes it from other organizations: and (a) embodies members' collective perceptions about their organization with respect to such dimensions as autonomy, trust, cohesiveness, support, recognition, innovation,

TABLE 2. Gouldner's Three Patterns of Industrial Bureaucracy

Mock Organization	Representative Organization	Punishment-Centered Organization
1. Rules are neither enforced by management nor obeyed by workers	1. Rules are both enforced by management and obeyed by workers	1. Rules are either enforced by workers or management and evaded by the other
2. Usually entails little conflict between two groups	2. Generates few tensions but little overt conflict	2. Entails relatively great tension and conflict
3. Joint violation and evasion of rules	3. Joint support of rules	3. Enforced by punishment

and fairness; (b) is produced by member interaction; (c) serves as a basis for interpreting the situation; (d) reflects the prevalent norms, values, and attitudes of the organization's culture; and (e) acts as a source of influence for shaping behavior."[10]

Shannon draws a distinction between "workplace organization," which refers to policies, procedures, and attitudes at the worksite level, and "work organization," which is more applicable to individual characteristics of work, such as span of control and psychological demands.[16] Generally, call center workers work in small groups, but the work is individual. Each worker answers an individual call. Teams have been tried in this environment with mixed results.

Management Commitment and Employee Involvement

From a survey of 718 Canadian workplaces, Shannon showed that concrete demonstration by management of its concern for the workforce and greater involvement of workers in general decision-making resulted in lower lost-time frequency rates.[16]

Techniques exist to measure organizational commitment and management commitment.[13] Effective programs depend on the level of top management commitment: the stronger the commitment, the greater the potential for program success.[4] A questionnaire developed by Porter, Steers, Mowday, and Boulian has been used to measure the commitment of organizations.[12a]

The Learning Climate Questionnaire has been developed to measure what helped or hindered learning in the workplace.[3] If the rate at which an organization needs to change in response to changing demands is greater than the organization's capacity to learn or power to adapt to the unknown, it is postulated that the organization may not survive. The Learning Climate Questionnaire includes some of the following dimensions: management relations and style, time, autonomy and responsibility, team style, opportunity to develop guidelines concerning how to do the job, and contendedness. Some of these issues were included in the employee survey, especially those related to work values or job satisfaction.

Early intervention by medical professionals correlates with less overall time in rehabilitation and an earlier successful return to work.[5]

IMPORTANT DATA

It was possible to determine the date of injury and the date of injury report for employees in the company's customer satisfaction department for 1996. Using these data, Figure 2 was constructed to show the resulting effect on lost time or alternate work time. It is not possible to draw definitive conclusions based on a single year's data. Many lost-time injuries, which were a mix of acute and chronic injuries, were reported on the day they occurred. Figure 2 includes only data reflecting incidents for which there was a difference between report and injury date. In general, the early

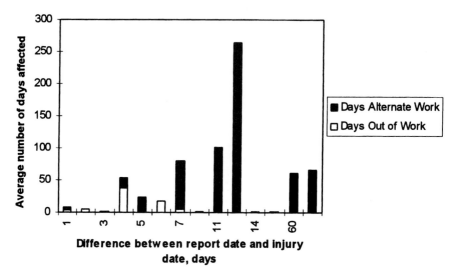

FIGURE 2. Effect of report date on recovery period.

intervention for injuries resulted in fewer days out of work and less time on alternate work.

An employee survey was conducted to determine the factors that would influence the early report of injuries.

EMPLOYEE SURVEY

Customer satisfaction employees at the two call centers were surveyed (Appendix). The survey was developed after discussion with health and management personnel at each location. The major elements of the survey included the following:

- Demographics—the number of temporary and permanent employees
- Job categories—customer representatives versus order representatives
- Reasons for not reporting pain
- Physical factors
- Work schedule
- Outside employment
- Work values

The author is aware of a similar survey conducted in 1991 at the company. This survey has been compared with the 1997 results (see below). The 1997 survey focused on understanding how injuries are reported and did not cover the design of the workstation in the same detail as the 1991 study.

Results

Table 3 summarizes the results of the survey conducted at the two call centers, site A and site B, during 1997.

A pain survey was included. Question 6 of the survey asked if the worker experienced pain at the end of the workshift. If they did experience pain, they were asked to indicate the body part that was affected. While fewer than 14% indicated pain at the end of a workshift, about half of the surveyed individuals completed the pain survey (Table 4).

TABLE 3. Summary of Results of Study Conducted at Two Call Centers in 1997

A total of 629 surveys were processed at site A and 683 at site B

Most temporary workers were order representatives and regular workers were customer representatives

Workstation preference was different at site A and site B

Work schedules were similar

Higher use of physical therapy at site B than site A

Most important reason for not reporting was more restricted work hours and fear of job loss

Pay and opportunity to advance were valued most for work at the company

97% of employees consider the company a safe place to work

TABLE 4. Overall Results of Pain Survey

A total of 334 surveys completed at site A and 353 at site B

About half of survey respondents completed the pain survey

Neck, shoulder, and low back pain accounted for about 44% of reports

The results of the 1997 and 1991 surveys were compared. For questions on the kind of workstation normally used, the 1991 results reflected the recent installation of adjustable workstations. By 1997, workers had used the various designs and were accustomed to changing and adjusting workstations to fit individual work modes. This is reflected in the fact that standing was expressed as a preference only in the 1997 survey (Fig. 3).

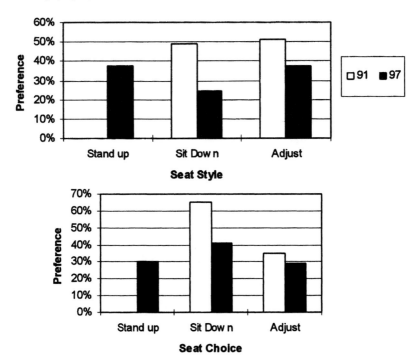

FIGURE 3. Workstation seating preference. *Top*, Call center site A. *Bottom*, Call center site B.

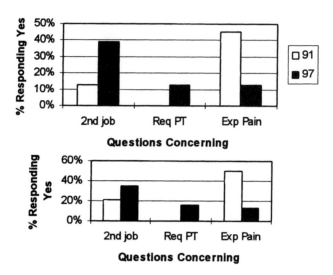

FIGURE 4. Employee responses to questions about outside employment, use of physical therapy, and pain experience. *Top*, Call center site A. *Bottom*, Call center site B. Req PT = require physical therapy, Exp = experience. (See questions 4–6 in Appendix.)

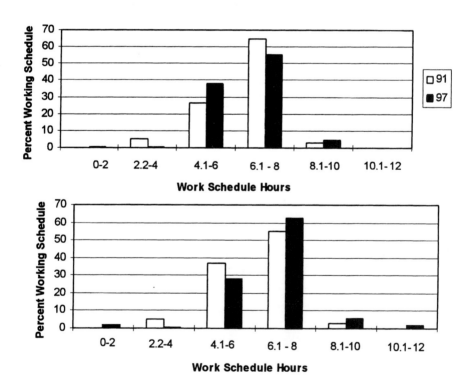

FIGURE 5. Preferred work shifts. *Top*, Call center site A. *Bottom*, Call center site B.

TABLE 5.   Reporting of Pain

Site A	No. Responses	%	Site B	No. Responses	%
When to report pain					
Immediate	410	65	Immediate	515	75
Next day	123	19	Next day	99	14
Week	71	11	Week	49	7
Never	14	2	Never	8	1
No answer	14	2	No answer	11	2
Multiple choice	1	0	Multiple choice	2	0
Reason for not reporting pain					
Restricted hours	157	32	Restricted hours	181	26
Fear job loss	136	28	Fear job loss	165	24
Time away from work	104	21	Time away from work	116	17
Promotion	72	15	Promotion	53	8
No Answer	14	3	No answer	129	19
Esteem factor	9	2	Esteem factor	3	0
Multiple choice	1	0	Multiple choice	37	5

A series of questions relating to outside employment, use of physical therapy, and pain experience were compared for groups surveyed in 1991 and 1997 (Fig. 4). It is of interest that more people reported a second job in 1997 than in 1991. There was no comparable question on physical therapy use in the 1991 survey.

Both surveys included a question on work schedules (Fig. 5). The number of hours worked was also an important factor. The 6- to 8-hour workshift was the most popular, followed by the 4- to 6-hour shift in site A in 1997, which had been the case at site B in 1991. This difference may reflect a change in the use of temporary workers at each location in 1991 and 1997.

Questions 7 and 8 concerned reporting of pain and were expected to give some insight into the reason early reporting is a problem (Table 5). Most respondents indicated that it was important to report pain immediately or the next day. The most important reason for not reporting pain was fear of restricted work hours or job loss.

Question 9 asked about work values (Table 6). Pay was the most important reason for working at both sites, but opportunity to advance was a close second at site B.

The pain survey (Table 7) compared favorably with actual injury experience for 1996 (Table 8). In the survey conducted in 1991, upper extremity and neck pain

TABLE 6.   Work Values

Site A	No. Responses	%	Site B	No. Responses	%
Reason for working at the company					
Pay	170	27	Pay	172	25
Other	113	18	Opportunity to advance	152	22
Opportunity to advance	104	16	Multi	114	17
Help people	89	14	Help people	99	14
Multi	73	12	Other	96	14
Contact coworker	67	11	Contact coworker	42	6
Not applicable	17	3	Not applicable	10	1

TABLE 7.   Pain Survey

Site A		Site B	
No. of Reports = 334	%	No. of Reports = 353	%
Neck	50	Neck	50
Shoulder	48	Shoulder	50
Low back	32	Low back	36
Wrists	25	Wrists	27
Eyes	20	Upper back	25
Upper back	18	Hands/fingers	19
Hands/fingers	18	Eyes	18
Head	15	Head	14
Hip/butt	13	Lower arms	12
Lower arms	12	Knees	12
Knees	10	Hip/butt	12
Ankles/feet	9	Upper arms	9
Elbows	8	Elbows	8
Upper arms	7	Ankles/feet	5
Lower legs	6	Ears	5
Ears	5	Lower legs	3
Thighs	4	Thighs	3

accounted for more than 50% of the pain at both sites. Table 8 shows that actual injuries were mostly in the upper extremities of the body. The neck, multiple upper extremity locations, and back account for many of the injuries resulting in lost time in 1996. The self-report of pain and the actual injury experience were comparable.

Discussion

The survey results did not yield many surprises. Fear of job loss as a reason for not reporting pain was hypothesized before the survey, and that—coupled with loss of time and loss of job advancement—were the major areas cited. Certainly, concentration of injury in the upper extremity compares with the self-report of neck and upper body pain.

Both in 1991 and 1997, 50% of survey respondents completed an anonymous pain survey indicating some level of pain. This indicated that much of the workforce was working in pain.

The question regarding work values resulted in a large number of people indicating that pay was a major reason for working at the company. Other surveys of private sector workers have indicated that compensation was not a major indicator of job satisfaction.[7]

Although 97% of the workers perceived the company to be a safe place to work, 50% were experiencing some work-related pain at the time of the study. The implications for reduced productivity and future injury at the company are significant.

Recommendations and Conclusions

The following recommendations are made as a result of this study.

1. Based on the high incidence of upper extremity pain, physical therapy and exercise routines should be tailored to the individual.

2. The effect on productivity levels for departments that have a high self-report of pain should be explored.

3. The fear of losing time or opportunity for promotion should be explored to determine if the fear is based in perception or reality.

TABLE 8. Actual Injuries by Body Part—1996

Body Part	Injuries	Lost Time Injuries	Body Part	Injuries	Lost Time Injuries
Head	1		Left arm	7	1
Ankle	1		Right arm	25	5
Left ankle	1	1	Elbow	2	
Right ankle	2	1	Elbow bilateral	1	
Left foot	1		Left elbow	5	2
Right foot	2		Right elbow	7	2
Knee	2		Hand, bilateral	3	1
Knee, bilateral	1		Hand	4	
Left knee	1		Right hand	11	3
Right knee	1		Upper multi	18	
Low multi	1		Shoulder	1	
Multi	25	10	Shoulder, bilateral	2	2
Neck	11	1	Left shoulder	7	
Other	7		Right shoulder	9	1
Back	24	2	Wrist	4	
Left hip	1	1	Wrist bilateral	8	
Upper extremity	1		Left wrist	6	
Arm	1		Right wrist	14	3
Arm, bilateral	3	2			

4. A reorganization of work to allow for job rotation and increased control may reduce psychosocial strain. Reorganization should not be undertaken without a thorough understanding of the workers' and supervisors' role. Specific training may be required to help with the transition.[8]

5. The supervisors' perception of the nature of their employees' jobs should be assessed to determine if the supervisors and employers perceive demands of the jobs differently. A difference in these perceptions can increase the pain experienced by the employee.[17]

6. Because the self-report correlates with actual pain experienced, a regular self-report survey should be instituted to monitor progress in this area.

This study has been able to identify important reasons employees are not reporting injury and pain at the catalog retailer. The company has taken many steps to understand the ergonomic stress in its workplace. It is clear that physical intervention alone will not solve the problem of increasing numbers of injuries at the call center. Attention to the psychosocial nature of call center work may lead to important clues in the etiology of musculoskeletal injury.

APPENDIX

Employee Survey Customer Satisfaction

Attached is a survey that is being given to every employee in customer satisfaction. We would appreciate your assistance by completing this survey and encouraging your fellow employees to complete the survey. This should be anonymous and finished in less than 10 minutes. Thank you.

1. Please circle whatever applies to you:

The Company Employment Status	Building	Job Status
Regular	Site A	Customer Rep
Temporary	Site B	Order Rep
	Site C	

2. What kind of workstation do you normally use?
   Stand up   ____
   Adjustable (active)   ____
   Sit down   ____

3. Please check the total hours per day you use a computer or write at the company.
   __ 0–2 hrs   __ 2.1–4 hrs   __ 4.1–6 hrs   __ 6.1–8 hrs   __ 8.1–10 hrs   __ 10.1–12 hrs

4. Do you have an outside job that requires using a computer, typewriter, calculator, cash register, or writing (please check)?
   Yes ____   No ____

5. Have you been in Physical Therapy in the last year?
   Yes ____   No ____

6. At the end of workshifts do you regularly experience pain? If yes, would you identify the body part affected on the chart on the reverse of this page?

   Yes ____   No ____

7. When is it important to report the pain?
   a. immediately   ____
   b. if it repeats the next day   ____
   c. if it lasts a week   ____
   d. never, it's part of the job ____

8. What would be the most important reason for not reporting pain?
   a. Fear of job loss   ____
   b. Fellow workers would think less of me   ____
   c. Fear of loss of promotion opportunity   ____
   d. Could result in restricted work hours   ____
   e. Takes time away from calls   ____

9. What do you value most about work at the company?
   a. Pay   ____
   b. Opportunity for advancement ____
   c. Chance to help people   ____
   d. Contact with coworkers   ____
   e. Other please specify _____

10. Is [the company] a safe and healthy place to work?
    Yes ____   No ____

REFERENCES

1. American Workers Under Pressure; Technical Report. St. Paul, The St. Paul Insurance Companies, 1992.
2. Arygis C: Understanding Organizational Behavior. Homewood, IL, Dorsey Press, 1960.
3. Brown AJ, Nixon S, Bartrum D, et al: Learning climate questionnaire (LCQ): Background and technical information. United Kingdom, Newland Park Associates Limited and Employment Service, 1993.
4. Gouldner AW: Patterns of Industrial Bureaucracy. New York, The Free Press, 1954.
5. Isernhagen SJ (ed): The Comprehensive Guide to Work Injury Management. Gaithersburg, MD, An Aspen Publication, 1995.
6. Karasek R, Theorell T: Healthy Work. New York, Basic Books, 1990.
7. Kohler S, Kamp J: American Workers Under Pressure. Technical Report. St. Paul, Minnesota, St. Paul Fire and Marine Insurance Co., December 1992, pp 12–13.
8. Levi's factory workers are assigned to teams, and morale takes a hit. Wall Street Journal, May 20, 1998.
9. Marmot MG, Bosma H, Hemingway H, et al: Contribution of job control and other risk factors to social variations in coronary heart disease incidence. Lancet 350:235–239, 1997.
10. Moran ET, Volkwein JF: The cultural approach to the formation of organizational climate. Hum Relations 45:19–45, 1992.
11. Most IG: The Quality of Workplace Organization and its Relationship to Employee Health [doctoral dissertation]. Lowell, MA, University of Massachusetts, 1998.
12. National Institute for Occupational Safety and Health: Study of Communication Workers at US West Communications. Cincinnati, NIOSH, 1992, HETA 89-299-2230.
12a. Porter LW, et al: Organizational commitment, job satisfaction, and turnover among psychiatric technicians. J Appl Psychol 59:603–609, 1974.
13. Reichers AE: Conflict and organizational commitment. J Appl Psychol 71:508–514, 1988.
14. Rodgers R, et al; Influence of top management commitment on management program success. J Appl Psychol 78: 1988.
15. Senge P: The Fifth Discipline. New York, Doubleday, 1990.
16. Shannon HS, et al: Workplace organizational correlates of lost-time accident rates in manufacturing. Am J Ind Med 29:258–268, 1996.
17. Warren N: The Psychosocial and Organizational Bases of Cumulative Trauma and Stress Disorders. Lowell, MA, University of Massachusetts, 1997.

CHARLES LEVENSTEIN, PhD, MSOH

ECONOMIC LOSSES FROM REPETITIVE STRAIN INJURIES

From the Department of Work
  Environment
University of Massachusetts
Lowell, Massachusetts

Reprint requests to:
Charles Levenstein, PhD, MSOH
Department of Work Environment
University of Massachusetts
1 University Avenue
Lowell, MA 01854

Musculoskeletal disorders resulting from cumulative trauma or repetitive strain can have an enduring disabling impact. Commonly, these repetitive strain injuries (RSIs) become worse over time, especially if hazardous exposure continues. According to Fine and Silverstein, "treatment is usually directed at two goals: to reduce inflammation or nerve compression, and to assist in the repair of any tissue damage. Symptomatic relief is provided by (1) the use of antiinflammatory medications, (2) rest (often facilitated by splints), and (3) application of heat or cold. Physical therapy techniques are used . . . Surgery, even in CTS [carpal tunnel syndrome, an RSI], may be ineffective if the worker is returned to the job without an effort to reduce occupational causes that are present."[1] For many individuals, RSI has an enduring impact on employment possibilities.

An economic approach is not useful or appropriate in evaluating the pain and suffering resulting from RSI. Frequently, the noneconomic aspects are the most significant for injured workers. The following accounts of injured office workers, offered as a response to an Internet query and discussion, illustrate these points.

The following narrative is provided by a library assistant:

I suffer from RSI. I was diagnosed approximately 3 years ago. At that time I had surgery for bilateral carpal tunnel. I now have many more problems with my wrists, arms, and hands. I was afraid of my employer and did not file for workman's compensation until after surgery.

My lifestyle changed greatly because of my income [loss]. Because of two surgeries within 6 months, my husband became my hands and arms. I am now able to work with lots of pain, but I will endure because that is my personality. I can't really afford to not work and enjoy my work. My husband still helps with all household duties.

... Many people asked what the scars are postsurgery. I used to say shark bite, shocked people quite a bit.

I now suffer from carpal tunnel, tendinitis in hands and wrists at times, and DeQuervain's. Life with RSI at times is unbearable but I [am] managing and trying to change my work habits and environment.

... [M]y salary was approximately $13,000 a year. I am doing the same job I was before the surgery. It is just a lot more difficult. I am making adjustments though to make the workplace more ergonomic and have had therapy and training on the computer to help. RSI affects every part of your life because your hands are involved, but you just tell yourself at least it is not life-threatening and go on.

Another office worker reports:

I will leave adding this up to you . . . . I was denied a raise, then laid off from work when I got the typing ban. I was out of work for 7 months, my new job entailed a 20% pay cut (and benefit cuts—the new job does not have a matched pension system), I spend $11,000 on a voice recognition system. I lost $25,000 worth of unvested employer contributions to my pension. I have had to pay my own health insurance to maintain coverage for some preexisting conditions.

I am in fairly steady pain, and thus irritable. I have had to stop playing my musical instruments (I haven't sold them off yet), and had to give up bicycle riding . . . .

Another office worker/computer user reported:

I have been treated for RSI (carpal tunnel & tendinitis) for the past 14 months. I have not had to take time from work, although I could have and probably should have. . . . I no longer play the violin or do hand sewing; the violin is a hobby, mending is not, I do pay to get that done, or have someone else do it. I very rarely prepare food that involves a lot of knife work, because it hurts. The food processor does most but not all that I'd like to do. I can't weed the garden or yard for more than a couple of minutes at a time. I can't turn the compost. I can usually carry my daughter, which I could not when my hand was really bad. I can't shuck corn, and I can't write at length with a pencil, although short periods of time are OK.

A computer science graduate student asks on an electronic bulletin board:

I'm a computer science Master student. . . . Because of the carpal tunnel syndrome I have, I am in the process of deciding whether I should just chuck computer science and change my profession. . . . If I'm very likely to be wrestled with wrist problem all my life, I might as well change my major right now while I'm still in school. My concentration is database, and as far as I know, every job I might have after getting my Master degree will require a fair amount of keyboarding.

The economic losses to impaired individuals as a result of loss of wages or salaries and of economically valuable household services is within the purview of the economist's expertise. Such calculation depends upon the degree of disability of the individual, which is established by medical and employment experts, as well as upon reasonable assumptions about the labor market, wage trends, mortality, and work life. This chapter reviews various considerations in the calculation of the economic loss of RSI, including lost employment income and the valuation of lost household services. The chapter does not consider economic losses to employers, such as workers' compensation premium costs and costs of training and retraining personnel. Nor does it deal with costs that society must bear, including income maintenance for disabled workers, and the provision of psychological or social work services for families of injured workers.

LOST EARNINGS

The first step in determining lost income is to estimate lost earnings from employment. Based on the wage or salary of the injured individual, we need to estimate the earnings the person would have made had he or she continued in the career in which he or she was engaged when becoming disabled. This estimate should include provision for fringe benefits, such as life insurance and health insurance, as well as required benefit programs, such as Social Security. Reasonable assumptions must be made about annual improvement factors (raises), promotions, periods of unemployment, and duration of work life. We can then calculate a total amount the worker might reasonably expect to have earned had no injury occurred. Similarly, we then calculate how much the worker with an indicated degree of disability is likely to earn in a lifetime in the labor market. If the worker is totally disabled, the full amount that the healthy worker would have earned is lost. If, on the other hand, the disabled worker is suited for some level of employment, again given assumptions (or actual information on current employment) about initial pay, improvement factors, possible promotions, fringe benefits, and work life, we can estimate total expected earnings for the partially disabled worker. Subtracting this estimate from the healthy worker estimate yields the amount of lost earnings from employment.

Earnings of Data Entry Personnel

This chapter focuses on estimating income loss related to RSIs among office workers using computers in data input work tasks. To illustrate the approach and to discuss the role of key assumptions in estimating earnings loss, we examine the considerations for keyboarding workers in the New York metropolitan area, as reported by the federal government. Although the wage rates will differ among regions, the results of this analysis can be extrapolated to other areas of the country.

WAGES AND SALARIES

The U.S. Department of Labor publishes area wage surveys for many metropolitan areas.[3] These reports include data on the weekly earnings of office employees with keyboarding responsibilities and information on wage trends and fringe benefits for office workers in general.

Table 1 presents information concerning average weekly earnings for secretarial and keyboarding occupations in the New York metropolitan area for 1990. In addition, wage data for clerical occupations not involving computerized data entry—file clerk and receptionist—are presented by way of contrast.

ANNUAL IMPROVEMENT

In estimating lifetime earnings for an individual, we start with an actual wage or salary but then must make assumptions about what the future would have brought

TABLE 1. Weekly Earnings of Office Workers (Range) in the New York Metropolitan Area, 1990

Secretarial and Keyboarding Operations		Nonkeyboarding Operations	
Secretaries	$564.00 (469.00–707.00)	File clerks	$273.00 (249.50–350.50)
Word processors	$477.00 (394.50–505.50)	Receptionists	$360.00 (not available)
Key entry operators	$372.50 (353.00–414.00)		

From Bureau of Labor Statistics: Area Wage Surveys, Selected Metropolitan Areas. Bulletin 3055-61. Washington, DC, United States Dept. of Labor, 1991.

TABLE 2.   Average Annual Pay in Seven Geographic Areas and Percent Change,
1987–1988 and 1988–1989

	Average Annual Pay			Percent Change	
Jurisdiction	1987	1988	1989	1987–1988	1988–1989
United States	$20,857	$21,872	$22,567	4.9%	3.2%
South Dakota	14,963	15,424	15,810	3.1	2.5
District of Columbia	28,477	30,253	32,106	6.2	6.1
New Jersey	23,842	25,748	26,780	8.0	4.0
New York	24,634	26,347	27,303	7.0	3.6
Metropolitan New York	25,976	28,104	29,208	8.2	3.9
Metropolitan Honolulu	19,718	21,196	22,399	7.5	5.7

Adapted from Statistical Abstract of the United States. Washington, DC, United States Government Printing Office, 1991.

if the worker had not become impaired. Because wages generally have been rising in the United States, we need to make assumptions concerning the rate of annual improvement for the particular worker. In part, an estimate might be made based on the experience of the worker in the past. However, because the gradual onset of RSI may have affected the worker's performance and earnings, it may be necessary to base the estimate on more general labor market trends.

The hourly earnings of all employees in nonfarm establishments in the United States rose from $2.09 in 1960 to $10.03 in 1990. In service-producing industries, the employment sector of particular interest in the investigation of data entry positions, wholesale trade hourly wages rose from $2.24 to $10.80 during the same period; retail trade wages, $1.52 to $6.78; finance, real estate, and related businesses, $2.02 to $9.99; and other services, $2.05 in 1965 to $9.86 in 1990.[6]

The percent changes in pay for all employees in the United States was 4.9% from 1987 to 1988 and 3.2% from 1988 to 1989.

However, substantial differences exist among geographic areas in the level of wages and salaries and in wage trends. In 1987, the average annual pay was $20,857 for the entire United States, below $15,000 in South Dakota, and above $28,000 in the District of Columbia. From 1987 to 1988, the average percent change in annual pay in individual states varied from a low of 0.1% in Alaska to a high of 8% in New Jersey. Table 2 illustrates the wide ranges in wages and salaries that should be taken into account in the projection of individual lifetime earnings and economic losses.

The U.S. Bureau of Labor Statistics' area wage surveys provide some indication of wage trends for office workers in manufacturing and other industries. Table 3 shows the rate of increase for an office worker in the New York metropolitan area for 1990; keyboarding employees are not singled out.

The calculation of wage trends by occupation, industry, and geographic area will suffice for estimation of lifetime earnings unless specific documents or procedures are available in specific cases. For instance, collective bargaining agreements or civil service procedures detailing wage or salary increases based on length of service can be used in particular cases. In general, no assumptions will be made about promotions, because there is no clear career path for many of the occupations of interest. However, in specific cases where career paths are established, such information may be used.

TABLE 3. Annual Rate of Increase for Office Workers in the New York Metropolitan Area, 1990

Job Category	Percentage Increase
All industries	6.2%
Manufacturing	6.8
Nonmanufacturing	6.0

From Bureau of Labor Statistics: Area Wage Surveys, Selected Metropolitan Areas. Bulletin 3055-61. Washington, DC, United States Dept. of Labor, 1991.

FRINGE BENEFITS

Fringe benefits represent a considerable proportion of employment costs for employers and a considerable portion of earnings for workers, and they have been increasing. While some benefits are legally required, others are optional for the employer. The U.S. Bureau of Labor Statistics estimates that for all employees, 28.6% of employment costs are attributed to fringe or nonrequired benefits. If total earnings—wages and benefits—represent 100% of employment cost for an American worker, 71.4% are accounted for by wages. Therefore, the benefits package is worth approximately 40% of wages (28.6/71.4). In estimating total earnings, we will use the 40% figure, but it is probably an underestimate of future costs because benefits have been rising at a faster pace than wages and salaries.

UNEMPLOYMENT FACTOR

In some projections of lifetime earnings, economists have argued that reasonable assumptions should be made about "normal" income loss from unemployment. A standard rate, related to the U.S. or relevant regional labor market unemployment rate, is used to reduce projected earnings. This approach is inappropriate for data entry and related computer operators, because such workers are among the employees most in demand in the U.S. The fastest growing occupations in the nation include medical secretaries, securities and financial services sales workers, travel agents, computer systems analysts, computer programmers, human services workers, and receptionists and information clerks.[6] It would be unreasonable to apply an unemployment rate for workers in general to this rapidly expanding occupational area.

WORKLIFE ESTIMATES

To estimate lifetime earnings from employment, it is necessary to make reasonable assumptions about the number of years that an individual will work. Men and women differ in life expectancy and in labor force participation. Differences also exist according to race and level of education. The most recent available analysis is

TABLE 4. Worklife Expectancy by Gender, Selected Ages

Age	Men	Women
25	33.1	24.0
35	24.5	17.6
45	15.7	11.1
55	7.8	5.2

From Smith SJ: Worklife Estimates: Effects of Race and Education. Washington, DC, United States Department of Labor, Bureau of Labor Statistics, 1986, Bulletin 2254.

TABLE 5.   Worklife Expectancy by Labor Force Status and Gender

	Men		Women	
Age	Active	Inactive	Active	Inactive
25	33.5	31.8	24.8	22.6
35	24.8	22.1	18.6	15.7
45	16.3	11.8	12.5	8.4
55	8.7	4.2	7.2	2.9

From Smith SJ: Worklife Estimates: Effects of Race and Education. Washington, DC, United States Department of Labor, Bureau of Labor Statistics, 1986, Bulletin 2254.

found in a 1986 publication of the U.S. Department of Labor, which is based in part on data from 1979–1980.[5]

The estimates in Table 4 are based on mortality tables developed by the National Center for Health Statistics and labor force participation rates from Department of Labor studies. Although the analysis attempts to identify gender, race, and education influences on length of work life, it does not show the impact of general employment and unemployment conditions in the economy or the impact of sex, race, and age discrimination on labor force participation. Therefore, using these estimates to project individual lifetime earnings of healthy workers may incorporate discriminatory bias into the estimates. Certainly, the inclusion of injured or disabled workers in the surveyed population reduces the worklife expectancy.

Table 5 shows the differences in worklife expectancy in 1979–1980 for active and inactive workers. At younger ages the differences are likely to be related to withdrawal from the labor force related to education for men and women and to childbearing for women. At later ages, however, the importance of illness and disability must increase, but no estimates of their relative impact are available. In addition, the availability of pensions and other benefits will have an impact on labor force participation.

It seems reasonable to assume in the estimation of lifetime earnings that healthy workers will work until age 65 unless specific information is available to suggest earlier retirement. For instance, the availability of a company pension plan enabling women to retire at 62 should be taken into account. On the other hand, it also seems reasonable to assume that disabled workers may have shorter worklife expectancy, as indicated by the data on "inactive" workers, i.e., workers temporarily out of the labor force for medical reasons but who later return as partially disabled employees are included in the inactive category. However, the worklife projections given in Table 5 suggest that only rarely do individuals work until age 65. Our preference is to rely on standard social/legal expectations about worklife rather than rely on figures that may mask important differences in labor market behavior among the healthy and the ill and among the rich, the working and middle classes, and the poor.

This chapter does not discuss the determinants of the degree of disability of workers with RSI. There are varying degrees of disability among such workers, ranging from total disability to temporary partial disability. Medical and other specialists will have to make that determination for individuals in light of the relevant labor market conditions.

New York Illustration: Retirement at 65

Data on office workers in the New York metropolitan area provided by the U.S. Department of Labor is used to illustrate the various considerations discussed above[3]

TABLE 6.   Lifetime Earnings of New York-area Office Workers,
after 20 and 30 Years of Employment, Assuming 6% Annual Increases

Job Title	Annual Earnings	Earnings, 1990–2010	Earnings, 1990–2020
Secretary	$29,328	$1,078,977	$2,318,671
Word processor	24,804	912,539	1,961,004
Key entry operator	19,370	712,622	1,531,392
File clerk	14,196	522,270	1,222,335
Receptionist	18,720	688,708	1,480,003

(Table 6). Suppose we hypothesize that three workers—a secretary, a word processor, and a key entry operator—all have RSI. The secretary is 45 years old and the others are 35 years old. Let us assume a 6% annual increase in pay for the secretary, who has been earning $29,328, the average for New York secretaries. Had she remained uninjured and continued to work until 65, she would have been paid $1,078,977 over 20 years. If she is totally disabled, all of those earnings will have been lost. If, on the other hand, she could still work as a receptionist, her loss in pay would amount to $390,268. The younger workers, if permanently injured at age 35, would have 30 years until projected retirement. A word processor whose job is reduced to that of a receptionist for 30 years would lose $481,001 in pay. The key entry operator, in this instance assumed to be only able to work as a file clerk for the next 30 years, would lose $409,056. These calculations do not include the value of fringe benefits.

Table 7 shows lifetime earnings adjusted to include the value of fringe benefits assumed to be worth 40% of pay. The injured secretary who becomes a receptionist would lose $546,375 in wages and benefits over 20 years. The word processor's loss over 20 years would be $673,401 if he or she were able to hold a receptionist's position. The file clerk who had formerly been a key entry operator will lose $572,679 in wages and benefits over 30 years. Table 8 summarizes income losses for keyboard operators who are totally disabled or able to work as a receptionist at selected ages.

New York Illustration: Alternative Retirement

In the previous illustration, the work lives of both healthy and impaired workers were assumed to continue to age 65. The U.S. Department of Labor's study of work life, however, shows that workers generally do not work until age 65, and it does not analyze the causes of leaving the labor market early. The averages may be brought down, for instance, by the inclusion of impaired or disabled workers, but we cannot tell by how much. Certainly, we do not want to penalize injured workers doubly by using worklife estimates that understate the figures for healthy workers

TABLE 7.   Lifetime Earnings and Fringe Benefits of New York-area Office Workers,
after 20 and 30 Years of Employment, Assuming 6% Annual Increases

Job Title	Earnings and Fringe Benefits, 1990–2010	Earnings and Fringe Benefits, 1990–2020
Secretary	$1,510,567	$3,246,140
Word processor	1,277,554	2,745,405
Key entry operator	997,671	2,143,949
File clerk	731,179	1,571,269
Receptionist	964,192	2,072,004

TABLE 8.   Hypothetical Wage and Fringe Benefit Losses Related to Repetitive Strain
Injury, Assuming Employment until Age 65 for Healthy and Injured Workers

| | Injured in 1990 at Age 45 | | Injured in 1990 at Age 35 | |
Job Title	Total Disability	Receptionist Option	Total Disability	Receptionist Option
Secretary	$1,510,567	$546,375	$3,246,140	$1,174,135
Word processor	1,277,554	313,362	2,745,405	673,401
Key entry operator	997,671	33,478	2,143,949	71,944

TABLE 9.   Worklife Expectancy for Selected Ages and Active/Inactive Status for White,
Female Office Workers in the New York Metropolitan Area

Job Title	Annual Wage	Age	Years of Remaining Work Life (Healthy)	Years of Remaining Work Life (Impaired)
Secretary	$29,328	45	12.5	8.4
Word processor	24,804	35	18.7	15.9
Key entry operator	19,370	35	18.7	18.9
Reception (impaired)	18,720	45	NA	8.4
Reception (impaired)	18,720	35	NA	15.9

NA = not available

TABLE 10.   Lifetime Earnings of White, Female, New York-area Office Workers, Using
Worklife Expectancy Tables Rounded to Nearest Year and Assuming 6% Annual Increases

Job Title	Annual Wage	Age	Earnings (Healthy)	Earnings (Impaired)	Loss
Secretary	$29,328	45	$554,299	$185,328	$368,971
Word processor	24,804	35	838,375	481,104	357,271
Key entry operator	19,370	35	654,706	481,104	173,602
Reception (impaired)	18,720	45	NA	185,328	NA
Reception (impaired)	18,720	35	NA	481,104	NA

NA = not available

and overstate the estimates for injured workers. The Department of Labor's study
does show future worklife estimates separately for individuals who were active and
inactive. Tables 9–11 assume that healthy workers were active and injured workers
were temporarily out of the labor force, or inactive, because of their disability.

The estimates developed in Tables 9–11 are based on the same hypotheses as
the previous New York illustration: a 45-year-old secretary, 35-year-old word
processor, and 35-year-old key entry operator—all women with RSI who are forced
to take employment as receptionists. Lifetime earnings including fringe benefits are
calculated and the losses shown in Table 10.

Summary: Lost Earnings

In summary, the following considerations must be taken into account in calculating lost earnings from employment:

1. Wage of healthy worker: actual wage
2. Annual improvement factor: regional or state estimate
3. Fringe benefit adjustment: 40% of wage
4. Unemployment adjustment: inappropriate for keyboard workers

TABLE 11.   Wage and Fringe Benefits Losses (Earnings Adjusted by 40%) of Repetitive Strain Injury-impaired Female Office Workers in the New York Metropolitan Area

Job Title	Earnings (Healthy)	Earnings (Impaired)	Loss
Secretary (age 45)	$ 776,019	$259,459	$516,560
Word processor (age 35)	1,173,725	673,546	500,179
Key entry operator (age 35)	916,588	673,546	243,042

5. Worklife estimates: assume retirement at 65 or use the United States Department of Labor's worklife estimate for active and inactive workers

VALUE OF HOUSEHOLD SERVICES

Economists have recognized that household production, although unremunerated, creates value and meets important needs. Household work includes "cooking, cleaning, washing, mowing, gardening, painting, and fixing."[2] The loss of such personal services through disability can be evaluated in financial terms. Essentially, we must estimate the average number of hours per week individuals devote to household production and find a market equivalent valuation (rate of pay) of that time. We must then make assumptions concerning "annual improvement" in the rate over an expected home work life. Then, separately from job market disability, we must have expert advice on the degree of impairment with respect to household activities for the individual and, from that, find the value of lost personal services.

Estimating Hours Devoted to Household Services

A study by Bryant et al. on economic valuation of household activities relies on survey data collected by the University of Michigan during 1975–1981.[2] Because the survey collected information on two-parent, or "intact families," the data probably greatly underestimate the time devoted by adults in single-parent households to personal service work. Table 12 shows their findings for married individuals by race and gender.

The data are presented separately by "black" and "nonblack" ethnicities, which does not seem to be a useful distinction for the purposes of measuring individual losses from occupational injury or disease. The categories are not valid ethnic, racial, or cultural divisions and may merely reflect unfairly discriminatory social situations. The "nonblack" estimate should be used, because it estimates majority behavior and includes a range of ethnic groups.

The loss of time to a family of an able-bodied mother is about triple the loss of a father. A reasonable estimate of the amount of household work by a single parent would be the sum of the hours for a married couple: about 40 hours per week in black families and 47.6 hours in nonblack families.

TABLE 12.   Median Hours per Week Spent by Married Individuals in Household Work

Sex	Ethnicity	
	Black	Nonblack
Males	9.64	12.75
Females	30.30	34.85

Adapted from Bryant WK, Zick CD, Kim H: The Dollar Value of Household Work. Ithaca, NY, Cornell University, 1992.

TABLE 13.   Estimated Weekly Hours of Household Labor for Full-Time Workers
(at Least 35 Hours per Week)

Number/Age	Married Men	Married Women	Single Parent
No children	12	22	34
One small child	20	35	55
Maximum (3+)	20	47	67

A key factor in determining the amount of household production is the number of children in the household. For men and women the time spent in household work for families with two working parents varies by number of children. The variation is considerable, suggesting that the number of children is a useful guide to estimating household work for an individual. The range for women is from a full-time female employee (working 35–40 hours per week) who spends 22 hours per week in household work to the mother of three children working more than 40 hours per week and spending 47 hours per week in household tasks. The range for full-time employed men (at least 35 hours per week) is from 12 hours for childless men to 19.6 hours for the father of four or more children.

Another important determinant of the amount of time an individual spends on household labor is the age of the children at home. Women in two-parent families who work full time spend 34.8 hours per week on household work if they have small children but 16.9 hours per week if they have no children or all their children are older than 18. Men in intact families range from 20 hours per week of household work when children are young to 9–12 hours in childless households or households with children older than 18.[2]

The final analysis must include reasonable assumptions about estimating the number of hours individuals spend in household labor based on sex, number and age of children, and marital status. It seems reasonable that the age of the youngest child should weigh heavily in these calculations (Table 13).

Estimating the Hourly Rate for Household Labor

To estimate the dollar value of household work, it is necessary to multiply the hours spent by a reasonable wage rate. Our approach is to use a rate that approximates the cost of hiring another individual to do the work. The rate will vary among geographic areas but is indicated by reported rates for common labor, custodial workers, or janitors. Table 14 shows the rates in manufacturing and nonmanufacturing industry for such jobs in metropolitan New York. Depending on the specific tasks, workers could be found at rates of $11–13 per hour. In addition, the hourly rate should reflect the additional 40% of employment costs attributable to fringe benefits. As was necessary in estimating earnings from employment, the labor rate

TABLE 14.   Common Labor, Custodial, and Janitorial Labor Rates,
Metropolitan New York, 1990

Job	Hourly Rate	Hourly Rate
	Manufacturing	Nonmanufacturing
Material handling/laborer	$12.86	$12.72
Janitors, porters, and clearners	11.02	11.07

Adapted from Bryant WK, Zick CD, Kim H: The Dollar Value of Household Work. Ithaca, NY, Cornell University, 1992.

for household work should be adjusted for an appropriate annual improvement factor. In New York, the rate of increase in 1990 for unskilled workers in all industries was 4.1%.[3]

Degree of Disability

In a manner similar to our calculations for employment income loss, a degree of impairment for household work must be provided by medical and occupational specialists. The degree of disability could vary from completely preventing an individual from engaging in household services to a much more limited disability, which may be nonetheless important.

Home Worklife Expectancy

Two main considerations play a role in determining home worklife expectancy and the intensity of homework: (1) life expectancy of the injured individual at the time of disablement and (2) age of children in the home at the time of disablement. Table 15 shows life expectancy for men and women at various ages based upon 1979–1980 data. Government analysts separately present data on whites and "others," a distinction that is not appropriate for our calculations. The figures for Caucasians should provide the basis for our calculations.

As indicated above, home work varies by sex and age of children. Our calculations also should reflect the amount of household service necessary as children mature and leave the home.

New York Illustration

Returning to our hypothetical injured workers in metropolitan New York, let us assume that the 45-year-old former secretary is divorced and her 20-year-old son is in college away from home. We calculate 34 hours per week of household services (see Table 13). Medical experts indicate that the level of household service-related impairment is 50%, so that she can only perform 17 hours of necessary home work. Let us apply the labor rate of $12 per hour, adjusted by a 40% fringe benefit factor, to equal $16.80 per hour. The annual value, then, of her lost capabilities amounts to $14,851. In New York, labor rates have been rising about 4% per year, but wage rates in general have been rising above 6%; we therefore estimate a rate of 5%. Her life expectancy is 35.6 years (see Table 15). If she lives 35 additional years, the lost services are worth $1,341,063.

Our second example was the 35-year-old injured word processor. Suppose that she is married and has a 3-year-old child. Table 13 tells us that, if healthy, she is likely to spend 35 hours per week in household labor in addition to her paid employment. Suppose she, too, has a 50% disability. Her life expectancy is about 45 years,

TABLE 15.   Life Expectancy in Years of Men and Women, 1979–1980 (Selected Ages)

	Men		Women	
Age	Caucasian	Other	Caucasian	Other
25	47.9	43.3	54.7	51.0
35	38.6	34.7	45.1	41.7
45	29.5	26.5	35.6	32.7

Adpated from Smith SJ: Worklife Estimates: Effects of Race and Education. Bulletin 2254. Washington, DC, U.S. Department of Labor, 1986.

but we cannot continue to estimate her household labor for the whole period as though her child remained 3 years old. We estimate, had she remained unimpaired by RSI, that over the next 15 years (since she has no other children) household labor would decline to 22 hours per week. Let us assume that while her child was in the household, she was only able to work 18 hours per week (losing 17 hours) and that in subsequent years she would work 11 hours per week, losing 11 hours. Her total loss over 45 years amounts to $1,647, 987.

Our third illustration is a 35-year-old disabled key entry operator, now capable of working as a receptionist. Let us assume she is married and has three children, ages 3, 6 and 12. Using Table 13, we estimate her household work at 47 hours per week when healthy. As her children age, her home work would have declined to 35 hours per week and then to 22 hours per week when her last child turned 18. If she is also impaired at a 50% rate, we would expect her to lose 23 hours of work per week for the next 6 years, 17 hours for the following 9 years, and 11 hours thereafter. Her total loss over 45 years amounts to $1,682,719.

Summary: Value of Lost Personal Services

In summary, estimating the economic loss from disablement that prevents an individual from fully engaging in household service requires attention to the following considerations:

1. Hours spent on household tasks depend on martial status, sex, and number and age of children
2. Rate of compensation depends on regional labor market rates for comparable labor and annual improvement factor
3. Life expectancy

VALUE OF ECONOMIC LOSSES

The money value of projected economic losses is calculated by adding the earnings losses from employment and the economic value of lost personal services. Table 16 show the losses of our three illustrative cases. Depending on which set of assumptions one makes, total losses can be estimated. Note that the value of lost personal services is considerable compared with wage losses; this is in part due to the selection of women for our illustrative cases.

To review the variety of considerations that should be taken into account in calculating lost earnings from employment, we base our calculations to start with on the actual wage of healthy workers. We then estimate an annual improvement factor from U.S. Department of Labor data available at the regional or state level. We assume a 40% fringe benefit adjustment to provide for additional nonwage mandatory and voluntary benefit programs. We have argued against an unemployment adjustment as inappropriate in the expanding market for keyboard workers. Our worklife estimates were calculated in two different ways, assuming retirement at 65 for healthy and impaired workers and, on the other hand, using U.S. Department of Labor worklife estimates for

TABLE 16.   Economic Losses of Hypothetical New York-area Office Workers
with Repetitive Strain Injury

Job Title	Lost Wages by Age 65	Lost Wages (Work Life)	Lost Personal Services
Secretary	$546,375	$516,560	$1,341,063
Word processor	673,401	500,179	1,647,987
Key entry operator	71,944	243,042	1,682,719

active and inactive workers. A critical input to these calculations is the degree of disability determined by medical and occupational experts.

In estimating the value of lost personal services, we have called attention to the number of hours spent on household tasks, depending on marital status, sex, and number and age of children. The rate of compensation that we assign to those tasks and those hours depends on regional labor market rates for comparable labor and the rate of annual improvement in wages in that market. Finally, life expectancy is a key factor. Reasonable assumptions about these considerations as well as those bearing on the wage loss calculation enable us to calculate acceptable estimates of the range of total losses.

CONCLUSION

Our hypothetical cases suggest that the economic losses to office workers can be considerable. The other side of the story is exemplified by the library assistant whose account we quoted at the beginning of this chapter. Her earnings were only $13,000 per year and, after a relatively brief period of disability, she returned to her previous position with no reduction in pay. She works in pain, and the real costs of her injuries are borne at home. Workers' compensation benefits, for which she was initially too frightened to apply, do not begin to compensate for her losses. It also is observed that the lower the wage of the injured office worker, the larger loom the losses in the home and quality of life. Failure to take into account the losses in household production is likely to bias regulatory analysis against the problems of low-wage workers.

REFERENCES

1. Andersson GBJ, Fine LJ, Silverstein BA: Musculoskeletal disorders. In Levy BS, Wegman DH (eds): Occupational Health. 3rd ed. Boston, Little, Brown, 1995, pp 455–487.
2. Bryant WK, Zick CD, Kim H: The Dollar Value of Household Work. Ithaca, NY, Cornell University, 1992.
3. Bureau of Labor Statistics: Area Wage Surveys, Selected Metropolitan Areas. Bulletin 3055-61. Washington, DC, United States Dept. of Labor, 1991.
4. Bureau of Labor Statistics: Employment Cost Indices and Levels, 1975–1992. Bulletin 2413. Washington, DC, U.S. Department of Labor, November 1992.
5. Smith SJ: Worklife Estimates: Effects of Race and Education. Bulletin 2254. Washington, DC, U.S. Department of Labor, 1986.
6. Statistical Abstract of the United States. Washington, DC, United States Government Printing Office, 1991.

EMIL F. PASCARELLI, MD

TRAINING AND RETRAINING OF OFFICE WORKERS AND MUSICIANS

From the Department of Medicine
Columbia University
New York, New York

Reprint requests to:
Emil F. Pascarelli, MD
228 West 11th Street
New York, NY 10014

The term "cumulative trauma disorders" (CTDs) describes the constellation of symptoms resulting from certain work-related activities that cause illness or injury. These activities are generally performed under conditions of sustained repetition, excessive force, or awkward positioning and are often associated with psychological stress and predisposing conditions such as poor posture, anatomic anomalies, and certain medical illnesses. Because so many factors are involved in their genesis, CTDs are generally poorly understood. This has resulted in the application of an array of terms in different disciplines and countries, none of which is truly a diagnosis. In Britain, Australia, and New Zealand, "repetitive stress injury" was commonly used until it was changed to "occupational overuse syndrome." "Repetitive strain injury" (RSI) is still in popular use in North America while "cumulative trauma disorders" is used in the scientific community. In Asian countries, "cervicobrachial disorder" seems to be preferred. Among musicians, "overuse syndrome" is commonly used. "Carpal tunnel syndrome" (CTS) is a specific diagnosis that is erroneously used as an overall term, particularly by surgical specialists who feel that CTS is one of the principal manifestations of this problem. Whatever else they may be called, CTDs are basically upper body soft tissue injuries that can involve nerves, muscles, tendons, ligaments, arteries, veins, connective tissue, and occasionally bone. Treatment of soft tissue injuries is primarily nonsurgical and is ideally a team effort involving a number of disciplines.

The association between repetitive work and illness dates back to the 18th century.[8] As the field of occupational medicine evolved, specific injuries relating to certain occupations were noted. Writer's cramp and telegrapher's wrist were reported in the late 1800s.[1] Later, workers such as carpenters and electricians were noted to have a high incidence of lateral epicondylitis from using screwdrivers and wire strippers. Specific soft tissue injuries were also described among musicians.[5]

To understand the etiology of CTDs, a distinction needs to be made between true occupational illness and work-related illness. In the latter, more than one factor is usually at play, as is the case with CTDs; in occupational illness, one specific cause is normally identified.

Injuries in white-collar workers doubled from 1960–1988, rising to 64.2 million.[1] This rise has been attributed to the advent of the personal computer in the early 1980s. Previously, CTDs were predominantly reported in industrial workers, but CTDs now account for about half of all occupational illness. From 1960–1988, the proportion of white-collar workers increased from 43.4% to 56% of the labor force, and the proportion of blue-collar workers decreased from 36% to 27.4%. Today, service industries employ about 75% of American workers (88 million–90 million).[1] These trends suggest that CTDs are likely to become more of a problem in the future if preventive measures are not taken.

CONCEPTS OF TRAINING AND RETRAINING

It was once common for students and office workers to be taught touch-typing and penmanship. Most people using computer keyboards have received little or no training in either skill. Musicians are trained by teachers who often have little education in the ergonomic and biomechanical aspects of musicianship. Music schools and conservatories have placed little if any emphasis on physical conditioning, just as physical conditioning has not been emphasized among office workers. It is therefore important to institute programs aimed at prevention and retraining to correct deficiencies that contribute to illness and injury.

There are two major components of training and retraining that act symbiotically: ergonomics and biomechanics. Ergonomics involves the study of how equipment can be fitted to the user to promote efficiency and comfort while reducing the likelihood of injury. Biomechanics is the study of how the body is used in its interaction with machines or equipment. Because each person has different physical characteristics, ergonomic and biomechanical factors have highly personal aspects. When training or retraining is undertaken, ergonomic and biomechanical aspects overlap. Therefore, proper training and retraining requires knowledge of both areas. The potential for inadequate solutions to work-related problems is increased if the trainer follows a "cookbook" approach. One must strive for comfort and safety through a knowledgeable application of ergonomic and biomechanical principles in the treatment and prevention of work-related disorders.

Ergonomics is a rapidly expanding field that has applications in the many areas where people work and perform activities of daily living. Trained ergonomists often have engineering or management backgrounds, but occupational and physical therapists have begun to enter the field. Many companies with blue-collar or white-collar workers find it advantageous to employ ergonomists. Manufacturers, newspapers, and banks and other service companies are able to make ergonomic adjustments to equipment and workstations that are often beneficial in preventing illness. Unfortunately, sometimes because of company policy, ergonomists may work in isolation without developing a relationship with other health care providers who can complete a team. A team approach is ideal for prevention and treatment. If only the ergonomic aspect is applied, it alone will not be enough.

Ergonomic design based on scientific principles has been beneficial in reducing the incidence of illness and injury. However, some principles that are claimed to be ergonomic are not based on the study of human anatomy or physiology.[3] For instance, a wide variety of office equipment is advertised as being able to prevent or cure various ailments.

Many musical instruments are ergonomic disasters, but attempts to modify or change them meet resistance based on old and strong traditions.

Blue-collar workers who perform more lifting and engage in heavy loading of the musculoskeletal system are more likely to benefit from ergonomic changes in tools and in the height and position of workstations and assembly lines. These workers are more likely to develop low back problems and acute injuries, particularly as they relate to posture. It is important to teach these workers how to lift, bend, and position themselves and to train them to maintain good body strength and posture through stretching and strengthening exercises. Programs for analyzing and treating potentially harmful working conditions (work hardening) have been established at many companies and have been shown to be beneficial in reducing injury. Grading and categorizing the degree and intensity of work has moved from the area of research to practical application. Videotaping workers can help employers characterize various types of work.[7] Training classes are also useful to educate and retrain new and existing employees.

Office workers labor under slightly different circumstances than blue-collar workers. Although the work of a data entry processor might be termed "sedentary," it is far from it. Upper back, shoulder, and arm and neck muscles endure long periods of static loading, a condition that involves work associated with a marked diminution of blood supply to the muscles.[3] This occurs even when the hands are placed above the keyboard and no keying is taking place. Awkward positioning, such as dorsiflexion of the wrists that occurs when the forearms are placed on a table or on a "wrist rest" while keying, results in eccentric muscle contraction of flexors. Eccentric muscle contraction occurs when the muscle is lengthened and is particularly damaging to muscle fibers.[2] Another common predisposing factor is the gradual deterioration of posture with rounded or protracted shoulders and the forward head positioning that is common in office workers and musicians. This posture eventually can lead to nerve compression and traction in the neck, resulting in the headaches, chest pain, derangement of scapular movement with loss of shoulder range of motion, and peripheral nerve manifestations of the radial, median, and ulnar nerves. Further consequences include diminished muscle regeneration and sympathetic nerve dysfunction. The resolution of problems of this magnitude requires a team effort. No amount of technique retraining or ergonomic intervention is likely to bring about substantial improvement if a worker is deconditioned, has poor posture, or has an accompanying illness. The basic rules of training or retraining must include the steps described below. Diagnose and treat medical, postural, and soft tissue deficiencies with medical interventions, physical therapy, occupational therapy, and home exercise. If return to work is a viable option, it should be done gradually with specific goals and restrictions. Determining tolerance for work is critical because superseding that level of effort will result in a relapse of symptoms. However, a work capacity evaluation is of little value before such treatment has been completed. If return to work is contemplated, the ergonomic aspects of the work area must be addressed. For office workers, the main components include an adjustable chair, an adjustable pullout computer tray capable of angling, and an appropriate input device such as a mouse touch pad, roller ball, joystick, or foot pedal that is correctly located and positioned. Voice-activated equipment should be considered in certain circumstances, but some speech training is desirable before using it. The ergonomist should be in touch with a health care provider who can give additional insights into what might be necessary in a particular circumstance. Many injuries are related to poor technique. Proper technique is particularly important to computer users and musicians. Poor technique results in increased work and can be further aggravated by sustained work with insufficient rest breaks.[7]

In more seriously injured workers, eventual postural deterioration leads to weakening of the upper back muscles and loss of scapular control and shoulder range of motion, which sets off a chain of neuromuscular events. Shortening and tightening of the scalene and sternocleidomastoid muscles can result in a head-forward position, producing compression, and traction of nerves in the cervical and brachial plexuses.[10] Anomalies in the neck area such as fibrous scalene bands, cervical ribs, or elongation of the C7 transverse process and excessive bowing of the clavicle can predispose workers to cervical or brachial plexopathy, producing peripheral nerve symptoms such as cubital or carpal tunnel syndromes.[6]

ERGONOMICS FOR OFFICE WORKERS AND OTHER COMPUTER USERS

To prevent injury and to correct obvious ergonomic contributing factors in someone being treated for injury, it is important to teach workers about some of the criteria for judging the qualities of safe equipment at computerized workstations.

Seating

People who sit at workstations for long hours every day should be informed about what to look for in a good chair for use at home or at the office. A properly adjusted chair can help the user maintain good posture. Poor posture is one of the most common factors leading to the development of muscular imbalance and ultimately to the constellation of symptoms of CTDs. Height adjustability is a basic requirement of an office chair. The seat pan of the chair ideally should be adjustable so that it can tilt to allow the knees to be situated lower than the hips. This postural modification carries some of the body load to the feet, which should be placed firmly on the ground, and stabilizes the lower spine. With the thighs at a downward angle, there is more knee room for an adjustable keyboard tray to be installed at the workstation. many chairs do not have seat pan tilt, which requires that the pan be separated from the chair's back. If no seat pan tilt is available, a wedge-shaped pillow can be placed on the pan to produce the desired effect. The back of the chair ideally should tilt forward and backward to provide further support to the lower and mid spines. The back itself should not be so high as to obstruct scapular movement. Many people prefer chairs that have arms. However, if the arms are used as a support while keying, the work load is transmitted to the forearms, wrists, and hands, which prevents the shoulders and upper back from sharing the work load. Therefore, chairs with arms are not recommended, especially if they are not moveable and inhibit free arm movement. Finally, the chair should be easy to adjust, which is often not the case because the levers on many office chairs are often difficult to operate.

The Keyboard

Keyboards are too often placed at the standard desk height of 29–30 inches high, which is acceptable for handwriting but not for keyboard placement. When typists worked on standard manual typewriters, the desk upon which the typewriter was placed with 3–4 inches lower than the standard writing desk. When computer keyboards that are placed on a standard desk are too high for the user, an adjustable-height pullout keyboard tray is recommended. The tray also should be tiltable. With the far side of the keyboard slightly lower (negative tilt), the wrists can assume a neutral position, the shoulders are free to move, and the elbows can open beyond 90°. With the elbows in a more extended position, less traction is produced on the ulnar nerve.

An ergonomic evaluation should document workstation measurements so that workers will know how to properly adjust their workstations wherever they go.

The height of the screen is adjusted for comfort, which usually means that the eyes fixed at the center of the screen are about 15–20° down from a gaze aimed at the top of the screen. Proper optical correction should not be forgotten as another important component of comfort. Special bifocals may be necessary.[7]

Many so-called "ergonomic" keyboards have been introduced and then removed from the marketplace for reasons including lack of consumer interest or price. The standard QWERTY-configured keyboard is still the norm. Attempts have been made to popularize the so-called DVORAK configuration, which groups the most frequently used keys in the central portion of the keyboard.

Keyboards with more function keys can place the user at greater risk, especially if his or her technique is poor. Splitting the keyboard has become a popular adaptation since it has been recognized that most persons tend to put their wrists into ulnar deviation on the standard keyboard. Our observations have shown that this tendency is increased in pronation, when the carrying angle at the elbow is more than 10°. Therefore, we recommend an adjustable or fixed split keyboard for these workers.

Laptop Computers

The tendency to place the wrists in ulnar deviation is enhanced by the cramped nature of the laptop keyboard. Visualizing the screen also presents the risk of excessive neck flexion. When possible, the screen should be placed at a comfortable height and a standard keyboard plugged into the laptop. The laptop's keyboard also can be placed on a pullout tray. Ironically, many people who demand an ergonomically sound set-up at work use a laptop at home on the kitchen or dining room table with inappropriate seating or use it in cramped positions such as in an airplane seat.

Laptops have various input devices. Touch pads and roller balls are the most common and are centrally or laterally positioned. Some have tiny joysticks buried among the keys. The close proximity of the input device to the keys is advantageous because it diminishes but does not eliminate the problem of excessive wrist motion in ulnar or radial deviation. Because the laptop is one integral unit usually including batteries, it is heavy and might be difficult for someone with CTDs to carry.

Input Devices: The Mouse, Touch Pad, and Roller Ball

With the proliferation of window programs, the input device has become a more frequent cause of problems. The mouse comes in a variety of sizes and shapes. The placement of the mouse is critical; it is often placed too high and too far away from the user. The idea is to get the mouse close to and at the same level as the keyboard to avoid problems related to stretching and static loading. People often squeeze the mouse too hard, which can cause thumb tendinitis. Special multiple functions, such as the puck used by graphic artists and architects, place the user at greater risk.

Many typists make little use of the number pad on the keyboard. Several companies make a metal cover on which you can rest the mouse or touch pad. This cover can be positioned over the number keys and slid away if the number pad is needed.

The touch pad is a comfortable and flexible alternative to the mouse. If stroked gently and properly positioned, it can alleviate some of the gripping problems associated with the mouse. Another advantage is its versatility of placement. Avoiding finger tension when using this device is important. Not everyone likes the feel of a touch pad, but most users, particularly laptop users, find it to be a comfortable input device.

Roller balls come in many sizes, ranging from the size of a cherry on some laptops to the size of a billiard ball as a separate device. Placement is important so that an ergonomically comfortable hand position can be achieved.

THE ERGONOMICS OF MUSICAL INSTRUMENTS

Most musical instruments have long histories and traditions dating back hundreds of years. The way instruments are played is often carried over from generation to generation. Thus, the cello is played sitting and is positioned on the floor, and the violin and viola are held on the left shoulder. However, in dealing with discomfort and injury relating from the poor ergonomics of certain instruments, it is increasingly recognized that modifications to an instrument may be necessary to adapt it to a particular musician. The goal is to achieve greater comfort, less risk of injury, and a better quality of music—because the musician gains more muscle control. It is difficult to ascertain which instruments are the most dangerous because the number of injuries also relate to the total number of people who play the instrument. Because physical conditioning is not emphasized in the schools and conservatories, many musical students are poorly conditioned. They often spend longer hours practicing than athletes but forego the conditioning and rest intervals that athletes have.

Keyboard and String Instruments

Generally, little can be accomplished ergonomically to change the configuration of the piano or organ. Therefore, technique, postural training, and physical condition assume greater importance in prevention and treatment of injury. With the piano, the force necessary to play on the keys and the degree of tactile response of the keys can affect technique and the quality of the music. For this reason, pianists who can afford to do so transport their own instruments to their concerts. One concert pianist with small hands reportedly had a keyboard made with narrow keys to make it easier to perform octaves and other maneuvers. The organ presents its own set of ergonomic problems. The legs and feet of the organist are used as extensively as the hands and arms. Furthermore, there are usually several keyboards and numerous stops. Unlike piano keys, organ keys offer minimal tactile feedback. The organ bench may not be adjustable or only minimally adjustable, requiring a great degree of physical adaptability. An analogous situation can occur with electronic keyboards, which are sometimes played in tandem at different heights.

The guitar, banjo, violin, viola, cello, double bass, and many other string instruments present an array of ergonomic challenges, particularly with regard to positioning the instrument for comfort and ease of playing. With the guitar, one must consider the placement in both sitting and standing positions. The guitar often is held to the right side, causing flexing of both wrists. Technique training is very important, but should follow proper and comfortable placement of the instrument.

Placement on the shoulder is critical for the violin and viola. Most, but not all, performers use various shoulder rests. The main deficiency of these shoulder rests is lack of support in the area under the left clavicle, leading to instability and rocking of the instrument. This instability necessitates gripping the neck of the instrument with the left thumb to keep it from moving downward, resulting in a loss of dexterity and stability in the fingers while playing. The location of the chin rest also is important. Chin rests should be more centrally located on the body of the instrument. Greater stability makes squeezing the instrument by laterally flexing the neck unnecessary; thus, the common dermatitis known as fiddlers' neck is avoidable. Recently, an ergonomically modified viola was introduced that was more comfortable for the user but caused great discomfort among music traditionalists. Although such a modification is quite unusual, it nevertheless points to the problems associated with playing the instrument.

The cello is played sitting down, which puts the musician at risk for postural misalignment and low back pain. Therefore, attention must be paid to seating as well as positioning. Cellos come in different sizes and should be chosen for comfort based on the musician's physique. For players who prefer more horizontal positioning, floor pins that bend downward are available. Nonprotruding string keys are also available so the cello neck can be held closer to the left side of the face and neck.

People who play the double bass must be in exemplary physical condition or musculoskeletal problems eventually will ensue.

Height, size, and string tension are all factors that can be varied for comfort for musicians who play string instruments.

Wind Instruments

Wind instruments include the piccolo, flute, clarinet, oboe, bassoon, trumpet, French horn, saxophone, and tuba. Despite their variety, certain basic ergonomic rules apply. The wind instruments present the dual problems of embouchure and positioning. Embouchure is the relationship among the muscles of the mouth, pharynx, teeth, and other structures. Different injuries may result with each type of embouchure. Flutes and piccolos cause little soft tissue injury, but problems with posture and finger placement are quite common. Many flutes do not fit their users' hands and necessitate moving and extending two or more keys, particularly of the left hand. In addition, increasing the girth of the flute with clip-on "crutches" for more comfortable thumb placement may be necessary. Flutists occasionally develop focal dystonia of the orbicularis muscle, causing loss of lip control. Focal dystonia, also known as writer's cramp, can affect the hands and has terminated the careers of several famous musicians. Retraining usually fails.

The type of embouchure associated with the clarinet is unlikely to cause oropharyngeal injury, but a laryngocele or pharyngocele occasionally occurs in predisposed persons. Positioning problems are common with the clarinet. A common ergonomic problems is that the right thumb rest is usually set too low. The resulting adduction of the thumb causes the remaining fingers to lose dexterity. Levers and keys often need repositioning to bring the hand into position of function. This allows the fingers to assume a curved position, avoiding hyperextension and cocontraction of extensors and flexors. A neck strap with a wide band to support the clarinet is useful and is sometimes augmented by a chest post. Devices are available that support the instrument on the floor. The ergonomic problems with the clarinet also are present with the oboe, English horn, bassoon, and other double-reed instruments except that double-reed instruments can lead to high pressure in the oropharynx and, occasionally, deficiencies in control of the soft palate. Many musicians make their own reeds, which is a laborious process that may contribute to an existing injury.

With the trumpet, trombone, or French horn, soft tissue injuries to the orbicularis oris muscle can occur because the high pressures in the anterior portion of the mouth coupled with the external pressure of the mouth piece can cause focally diminished blood supply. Sustained playing of high notes in particular can result in tears or stretching of the upper or lower lip, a condition sometimes called the Satchmo syndrome. Oropharyngeal blowouts can occasionally occur in the larynx, pharynx, or cheeks. With the French horn, the thumb rest and the left hand levers are often too short, causing hyperextension of the fingers and anatomically inefficient posture. Traditionally, dimes have been soldered on the levers to correct this. With the tuba and similar instruments, physical conditioning is important. All of the wind instruments require good breathing habits, which should be an integral part of the training program.

Percussion Instruments

Percussion instruments include drums, timpani, cymbals, bells, chimes, xylophones, vibraphones, and other devices. A major problem in injured percussionists is their failure to integrate the activity of the shoulders, upper back, and arms into the process of percussing. Videotaped analyses show excessive wrist motion combined with little or no shoulder movement. This technique places an enormous burden on the relatively delicate forearm muscles and the intrinsics of the hand, especially in drummers who grip the sticks tightly. Rock drummers seem more prone to tight gripping. Lack of proximal body use is the sports equivalent of a baseball pitcher trying to throw a baseball 90 miles per hour by flicking his wrist. This problem can be overcome primarily by conditioning and retraining, which implies a change in technique. Abducting the arms away from the body will promote a smoother integration of body musculature.

Every musical instrument has its own potential ergonomic problems, which should be addressed where possible by a careful analysis of the instrument and its relation to the musician's body.

BIOMECHANICAL TRAINING AND RETRAINING OF COMPUTER USERS

Training in the technique of proper keying is a lost art. Although manual typewriter technique and handwriting are rarely taught in schools, technique training is even more important today because the inherent characteristics of the computer keyboard and its associated input devices all but encourage poor technique. One of the most common problems in an office is the placement of the keyboard on a standard height desk. The keyboard is often inclined using legs at the far end to imitate the stepped effect of the keyboard on a manual typewriter. This "ramp" encourages the user to extend the wrists while the forearms rest on the table. Under these circumstances the work load rests entirely with the forearm muscles. By extending the wrists, the forearm flexor muscles are stretched, resulting in harmful eccentric muscle contraction. The flexor tendons are no longer moving in a straight line but must now bend around the sheath's wrist, creating greater friction and shear at the tendon sheathes and pulleys. The main pulley to be affected is the transverse carpal ligament. The keyboard layout also encourages the user to place the hands in ulnar deviation, as discussed above. Therefore, the first element of training is to establish a neutral position of the hand with a straight line from forearm to the top of the middle finger. The fingers are held in a natural slightly curved position, and the arm "floats" above the keyboard even if there is a wrist rest. This also applies to the use of laptops, which have a flat surface in front of their keyboards. In essence, we should be looking for a straight line from the forearm to finger tips, no extension or exaggerated flexion of the wrist, and a hand that floats above the keyboard. Such positioning will prevent hyperextension of the fingers while reaching function keys. The back and shoulders should carry the entire hand to these keys. The mouse should be gripped lightly and at the same level as the keyboard; gentle pressure should be applied to click, and the hand and the forearm should be anatomically aligned. The touch pad should be stroked lightly and the roller ball stroked gently. The thumbs should be relaxed and not stick upward. Many people do this with one hand to avoid striking the space bar.[9] The user should be instructed to use both thumbs for this activity. In two or three 40-minute sessions, ergonomists and biomechanical trainers should observe for deficiencies, work on correcting them, and analyze use of the pen during handwriting. For workers who grip their pens too tightly or use a pen input device, a sponge curler expander placed on the pen shank may be necessary to loosen the grip.

BIOMECHANICAL TRAINING OF MUSICIANS
The biomechanical training of musicians brings up some interesting philosophical issues. Biomechanical retraining for musicians is best done by another knowledgeable musician and would be an appropriate part of the curricula of music schools and conservatories.

The training and retraining of musicians is complex. However, once the ergonomic issues of each instrument have been addressed and a physical conditioning program established, biomechanical rehabilitation can begin. Some basic rules need to be followed, including:

1. The musician should be comfortable with his or her instrument, teacher, and audience. Because performance anxiety is common, psychologic intervention may be necessary.

2. The hands, forearms, arms, shoulders, back, and the entire body should perform synchronously with as little isolation of particular muscle groups as possible.

3. Postural misalignment will need correction, and proper use of the hands should be accompanied by a gradual changing style or repertoire.

4. A "carry over" of technique deficiencies can exist, which also may need retraining. Carry-overs include deficiencies in handwriting, typing, and activities of daily living.

5. People who have developed focal dystonia will need long-term corrective treatment. Focal dystonia of the mouth muscles may require a change to a different embouchure, such as from the flute to clarinet.

6. Videotaping is an essential part of biomechanical training because (1) the original status of the typist or musician becomes an important point of reference (2) it allows technique and positioning to be analyzed in stop motion or frame-by-frame analysis, and (3) it can demonstrate needed changes to the musician, who is often surprised when observing himself. Follow-up videos can be compared with initial takes to document progress. Videotaping is also useful for evaluating computer keyboard technique.

In a recent study of injury, about 90% of 50 pianists had a characteristic postural misalignment consisting of head-forward positioning, rounded shoulders, loss of scapular function, and rigidity of the cervical and thoracic spines. This positioning resulted in a high incidence of brachial plexopathy manifested by pain, loss of dexterity, and many other neuromuscular manifestations.[4] The pianists tended to compensate for not using their shoulders by using their hand and forearm muscles excessively. Associated problems included ulnar deviation, wrist extension, and hyperextension of the fingers. In such instances, biomechanical retraining consists of different use of shoulder musculature, change of fingering, and reorganization of the repertoire.

With string instrument players, the situation is more complex because the aberrations of technique are often different in each hand. Instrument positioning plays a major role in the rehabilitation process; once positioning is corrected, technique tends to improve. A total physical conditioning program is necessary to enable the musician to sustain proper posture, gain greater strength, and follow prescribed measures.

In users of woodwind and brass instruments, correction of biomechanical deficiencies will often lead to greater comfort. This is particularly true of embouchure problems, where excessive practicing, limited rest breaks, and poor breathing habits are potential sources of difficulty.

Because percussionists engage in more upper- and lower-body activity than most musicians, it is important for them to engage in a continuing conditioning program. Percussion instruments should be arranged low enough to allow full upper body movement and comfort. Posture and physical condition play a critical role in determining whether a percussionist is successful in terms of his playing ability as well as his appearance as a performer.

REFERENCES

1. Bureau of Labor Statistics: Occupational Injuries and Illnesses in the United States, 1992. Washington, DC, U.S. Dept. of Labor, 1994, government document L 2.2: OCI/153.
2. Fridén J, Sjöström M, Erblom B: Myofibrillar damage following intense eccentric exercise in man. Int J Sports Med 4:45–51, 1983.
3. Grandjean E: Ergonomics in Computerized Offices. London, Taylor & Francis, 1987.
4. Hsu YP: An analysis of contributing factors to repetitive strain injury (RSI) among pianists [doctoral dissertation]. Ann Arbor, MI, Teachers College, Columbia University, 1997.
5. Lederman RJ: Thoracic outlet syndromes: Review of the controversies and a report of 17 instrumental musicians. Med Probl Perform Art 2:87–91, 1987.
6. Pascarelli EF, Kella J: Soft-tissue injuries related to use of the computer keyboard: A clinical study of 53 severely injured persons. J Occup Med 35:5, 1993.
7. Pascarelli EF, Quilter D: Repetitive Strain Injury: A Computer User's Guide. New York, Wiley & Sons, 1994.
8. Ramazzini B: De Morbis artificum diatriba, Disease of workers, 1713 [translated by Wilmer Cave Wright]. Chicago, University of Chicago Press, 1940.
9. Roos DB: Overview of thoracic outlet syndromes. In Machleder HI (ed): Vascular Disorders of the Upper Extremity. Mt. Kisco, NY, Futura Publishing, 1989.
10. Schwartzman RV: Brachial plexus traction injuries. Hand Clin 7:547–555, 1991.

INDEX

Entries in **boldface type** indicate complete chapters.

Keyboarding, 1–2, as musculoskeletal disorder
  cause. *See also* Video display terminals
  eccentric muscle contraction associated with,
    165
  epidemiologic studies of, 19–28
    individual risk factors in, 32–33
    physical risk factors in, 28, 32–33
  force and repetition parameters of, 8–9
  relationship to duration of typing, 29–30
  relationship to nonneutral joint postures, 31–32
  relationship to posture, 51, 75
  relationship to typing speed, 30
  relationship to work-related cycles, 30–31
  as repetitive strain injury cause, 4, 85, 92
    income loss related to, 149–157
  among telegraphers, 19–20, 23

Labor unions, 64, 68, 70, 85
Levator scapulae muscle, overuse of, 41, 42
Lighting
  ergonomically-correct, purchasing strategy for,
    133
  as eye complaint cause, 127–128, 129–130
Loading, static, 165
Los Angeles Times, 21, 22
Low back disease
  biomechanical factors in, 4
  degenerative spinal disease-related, 7

Mammoplasty, reduction, 53
Management, scientific, 66
Management personnel, participation in
  ergonomics programs, 132–133
Manufacturing industry workers, carpal tunnel
  syndrome in, 39
Medial antebrachial cutaneous nerve, in ulnar
  nerve decompression, 54
Median nerve, compression of, 41
  provocation testing for, 45, 46
  sites of, 42
Mononeuritis, 88
Muscle
  abnormal posture-related imbalance of, 41,
    42
  injury mechanisms in, 84–85
Muscle fiber, gender differences in, 120–121
Muscle strengthening exercises, as nerve
  compression syndrome therapy, 53
Muscle strength testing, 47
Muscle stretching exercises, as nerve compression
  therapy, 51–52
Musculoskeletal disorders. *See also* Cumulative
  trauma disorders; Repetitive strain injuries
  costs of, estimation of, 77–78
  definition of, 17–18
  early diagnosis of, effect on long-term
    rehabilitation, 137, 139–140
  prevalence of, 17
  symptoms of, 21
Musical instruments, ergonomics of, 165,
  168–170

Musicians
  biomechanical training and retraining of,
    171–172
  overuse syndromes in, 5–6
Myalgia
  anthropometric factors in, 33
  muscle pathology in, 85
  nonneutral joint posture-related, 31
  in telegraphers, 19–20

National Commission on State Workman's
  Compensation Laws, 70
National Institute for Occupational Safety and
  Health (NIOSH), 6–7
  musculoskeletal disorder epidemiologic studies
    by, 19, 20–21, 22, 28
  psychosocial risk factor identification in,
    34–35
  occupational exposure model of, 8
Neck pain, in office workers
  ergonomic factors in, 125, 126, 127, 133
  in video display terminal workers, 116–119,
    120, 121–122
Nerve compression, **39–59**. *See also* specific
  nerves
  causes of, 39
  chronic
    double crush theory of, 44, 45
    evaluation of, 44–48
    histopathology of, 41–42, 43
    nonsurgical management of, 48–53
    surgical management of, 41, 53–56
    symptoms of, 41, 44–45
  provocation testing of, 45–46, 47, 48
Nerve conduction studies, for carpal tunnel
  syndrome diagnosis, 18, 89
Neuropathy, peripheral, vibration-related, 8
Neuroplasticity, 87
Newspaper industry personnel
  musculoskeletal disorders in
    epidemiologic studies of, 21–22, 24–25
    relationship to work postures, 32
    upper-extremity disorders in, 2–3
  video display terminal-related health risks of,
    69–70
New York City metropolitan area
  household services labor rates in, 158–159
  office workers in
    earning trends among, 152, 153
    musculoskeletal disorder cross-sectional
      studies of, 21, 22
    repetitive strain injury-related economic
      losses by, 155–157, 160
NIOSH. *See* National Institute for Occupational
  Safety and Health
Nurses, in ergonomics programs, 76

Obesity, as nerve compression risk factor, 18,
  53
Occupational illness, differentiated from work-
  related illness, 164